Medical Law Handbook

Medical Law Handbook

RAJ MOHINDRA

MA (Cantab) BM BCh (Oxon) MRCP(UK)
Barrister-at-Law (non-practising) of the Inner Temple
MA (King's London) (Medical Law and Ethics)
Consultant Cardiologist

Radcliffe Publishing
Oxford • New York

Radcliffe Publishing Ltd
18 Marcham Road
Abingdon
Oxon OX14 1AA
United Kingdom

www.radcliffe-oxford.com
Electronic catalogue and worldwide online ordering facility.

British Library Cataloguing in Publication Data

A catalogue record for this book is available from the British Library.

ISBN-13: 978 184619 067 4

Typeset by Pindar NZ (Egan Reid), Auckland, New Zealand
Printed and bound by TJI Digital, Padstow, Cornwall, UK

Contents

About the author

Raj Mohindra graduated from Cambridge where he studied pre-clinical medicine and law. Having determined to combine medicine and law he proceeded to complete the Bar exams before moving to Oxford to complete his clinical medical training. After MRCP he continued in medical training, first in general medicine then cardiology. During this time he completed a Masters in medical law and ethics at King's College, London.

He has just completed his medical training and is currently working as a consultant cardiologist within the NHS in the North East of England.

His interest lies in the overlap of medicine law and ethics as it impacts upon the daily practice of medicine as well as in the daily practice of clinical medicine itself.

*This book is dedicated to my wife, my parents, my brothers and sister
and to my gloriously burgeoning number of nieces and nephews*

List of figures and tables

FIGURES

TABLES

List of legal references

Page numbers in **bold** indicate summaries of cases.

CASES

STATUTES

LIST OF LEGAL REFERENCES

STATUTORY INSTRUMENTS

ECHR AND EUROPEAN LAW

OTHER AUTHORITIES

Australian cases

Canadian cases

USA cases

LIST OF LEGAL REFERENCES

1 Introduction

1.1 AIMS

1.1.1 Modern medicine requires working within an evidence based framework. It also requires working within a rapidly evolving and important legal framework. The purpose of this book is to provide an accessible resource for busy medical professionals. It is designed to expose the important principles and structures of the law that surround modern medical practice in a way medical professionals are familiar with, i.e. by looking at the facts of interesting cases.

1.1.2 The text assumes no knowledge of law and is extensively cross-referenced. The facts and results of the important cases cited are set out and integrated into the text. The cases have been selected to be illuminating, interesting and, I hope, entertaining.

1.1.3 The medical factual details that are often frustratingly missing from legal textbooks are retained. The point is to locate the cases not just on the legal maps but also upon the medical maps. Because of the burgeoning size of the text, ethics has not been considered.

1.1.4 For the same reason, a degree of selection of topics and legal materials has been necessary. I have focused on core concepts in important everyday topics. For efficiency, the aim has been exposition rather than discussion.

1.1.5 Like medicine the law is a dynamic structure. I have endeavoured to state the position as it stood at 31 October 2007. Given the inevitable delay between this date and the date of publication, together with its nature, this book should not be relied upon to provide solutions to individual problems. The aim is to illustrate and illuminate.

1.2 THESIS

1.2.1 Legal principles seek to locate and protect, to varying degrees, certain critical **interests** we all possess. They must also deal with situations where these critical interests conflict. Key critical interests include the interest in life, the interest in being free from unjustified physical interference, and the interest of privacy.

1.2.2 The thesis of this book is that these critical interests form a deep structure from which we can source virtually the entire legal framework. Discussions of the more superficial legal structure of rights and duties should take into account this deep structure.

1.3 SOME CORE PRINCIPLES

1.3.1 The core mechanics of the law are integrated into the text at appropriate points. However, as part of this introduction we will now cover a few broad concepts needed to unlock the text most effectively.

1.3.2 The idea of a **duty of care** (*see* Section 9.1) is more than a moral obligation. In this context, a duty of care is a legally enforceable obligation often mirrored by a corresponding right. The question is not just is there a moral obligation but, given this moral obligation, should the law impose a sanction for the breach of this obligation?

1.3.3 **Rights** are also legally enforceable obligations that can simply be the correlates of duties, e.g. the patient's right to care correlates to the medical professional's duty to treat. However, rights can stand free from correlative duties by resting wholly upon an underlying interest, e.g. a right to life of Tony Bland in the *Bland* case (*see* Section 19.10.1).

1.3.4 Two key principles which I believe should be developed and then incorporated into medical decision-making methods are legal case-based reasoning and the doctrine of precedent. Together, the cumulative decisions made by judges form a set of rules called **case-law** or **the common law**.

1.3.5 **Legal case-based reasoning:** Cases are decided with the underpinning reasoning expressed in the judgments. Where conflicting, these decisions and their reasoning are considered in subsequent cases in the light of new facts and the reasoning developed as necessary. A rational framework emerges from this dialectic which forms the reasoned basis for the present decision. It is this framework that we will be exploring.

As new cases arise this framework is continually refined and extended (for an example *see* paras. 13.2.7–13.2.18).

1.3.6 **The doctrine of precedent** (*stare decisis*): The principle of binding precedent holds this common law framework in existence and allows it to maintain a coherent evolutionary direction. Binding precedent means that the previous decisions of higher courts bind the choices available to the lower courts. By a principle of logic, the court making the decision itself is also bound by its own decisions.[1] The only exception to this latter rule is the House of Lords itself, which on occasion has overruled its own previous decisions.[2]

1.3.7 The case-based nature of the common law permits a rich base of principles and factual elements to be mined and then made coherent through subsequent decisions made in accordance with the principle of justice. By operation of the doctrine of precedent the framework that emerges must inevitably be internally consistent.

1.3.8 **Acts of Parliament** are the rules made by Parliament that carry the force of law. Within the United Kingdom constitution Parliament is sovereign. Therefore, where both common law and statutory rules operate, the rules made by Parliament prevail. Human rights law (for approach, *see* Sections 2.5.6 and 2.5.7) and European law are introduced as necessary into the text.

1.3.9 **Judicial review** is one way to challenge a decision made by Government and its related bodies. The important point to note is that judicial review does not consider whether the decision reached was right or wrong. It only tests if the decision was made in a correct manner. Additionally, there is an area of discretion within the power of decision-makers which the Court will not invade. If, however, the power of the decision-maker is exercised outside this area of discretion then the Court has the power to intervene.

1.3.10 Judicial review is a legal process whereby a decision can be challenged on three broad grounds:

(i) it was **procedurally unfair**[3]

---

1   *London Street Tramways v London County Council* [1898] AC 375.
2   Practice Directions. Judgment: Judicial decision as authority: House of Lords. [1966] 3 All ER 77.
3   *Council of Civil Service Unions v Minister for the Civil Service* [1984] 3 All ER 935.

(ii) it was so **unreasonable** that no reasonable[4] decision-making body could have made it,[5,6] or

(iii) it was **illegal**. Examples of the illegality challenge include:

    a) the power to make the decision did not lie in the hands of those who actually made the decision (*ultra vires*)

    b) the discretion was fettered, e.g. it was not a genuine exercise of discretion, simply the application of a blanket rule,[7] or the power to decide was inappropriately delegated

    c) irrelevant considerations were taken into account, or relevant considerations were not taken into account.[3]

1.3.11   Duties that arise generally within society without explicit agreement tend to fall under the heading of torts. A **tort** is a civil wrong. It usually arises as a breach of a legal duty owed between legal persons. Here we will encounter the torts of negligence and battery. Duties arising from agreements between legal persons fall into the **law of contract**. There are other sources of duties but the duties in tort and contract are the key ones we will consider here.

---

4   for consideration of reasonableness *see* Section 10.2.

5   *Associated Provincial Picture Houses Ltd v Wednesbury Corporation* [1947] 2 All ER 680.

6   *Rogers, R (on the application of) v Swindon NHS Primary Care Trust* [2006] EWCA Civ 392 (herceptin case); *see* also Newdick C. Judicial review: low-priority treatment and exceptional case review. *Med Law Rev* 2007; 15(2): 236–44.

7   *British Oxygen Company Limited v Board of Trade* [1971] AC 61, 625D per Ld Reid.

2 Confidentiality

2.1 INTRODUCTION

2.1.1 A duty of confidence arises when a medical professional receives information from a patient in the context of a professional relationship.[1] Here the medical professional has either implicitly agreed[2] that the information is confidential or knows, or should know, that that information is imparted in circumstances that impose a duty of confidentiality. This duty is not absolute, there are situations where such information can be disclosed.

Hunter v Mann [1974] 2 All ER 414, CA

X was involved in a road traffic accident but fled the scene. X was seen afterwards by a doctor (D) who treated X in his surgery and discovered that X had been involved in a road traffic accident. D advised X to attend the police station but X did not follow this advice.

The police sought the identity of X from D. D was made aware that the police alleged that X had been driving dangerously. D refused to disclose the identity of X in the *bona fide* belief that he was bound to hold it in confidence because he had come by the information through the doctor–patient relationship.

D was charged and convicted of failing to disclose the identity of X under s.168(2) of the *Road Traffic Act 1972*. He was fined £5.

D appealed on the basis that information acquired in the course of the doctor–patient relationship did not fall within the requirements of the *Road Traffic Act 1972* or that his professional duty of confidentiality to the patient meant that D did not have the power to disclose the information.

Held: Conviction upheld.
D did owe a duty of confidentiality to his patients. However this duty was overridden by the relevant provision of the *Road Traffic Act 1972*. D did have the power to disclose the information.

---

1   *See*, for example, para. 37 *A v General Medical Council* [2004] EWHC 880 per Charles J.
2   *Coco v A.N. Clark (Engineers) Ltd* [1969] RPC 41.

2.1.2   The legal structure surrounding questions of confidentiality has been in a state of flux since the introduction of the *Human Rights Act 1998*. To make sense of this process and to get a feel of its general direction, we will first look at this structure. This will also permit us to develop a deeper view of the concept of confidentiality. We will then move to consider the important exceptions to the broad rule of confidence that prevails in medical situations.

2.2   THE LEGAL STRUCTURE

2.2.1   The legal structure surrounding issues of confidentiality is an overlapping patchwork of case-law, Acts of Parliament (statute law) and human rights law. In addition, where relevant to the situation, particular codes of practice are considered when determining whether or not a breach of confidence has occurred.[3] This means that, for example, guidance from the General Medical Council is legally relevant when considering such issues. Like much of medical law, this structure is in a state of growth and evolution. We will consider initially how this development has progressed, then move on to consider the current position.

2.2.2   The basic interest protected in relation to personal confidences[4] is the **interest of privacy**.[5] This interest should not to be confused with the right to privacy.[6]

2.2.3   The interest of privacy is protected by the common law action for breach of confidence (*see* Section 2.4), the *Human Rights Act 1998*, in particular the Article 8 right to privacy (*see* Section 2.5), and the statutory provisions (*see* Section 2.11). Invasion of this interest of privacy is what provides the moral impetus for any legal action, although there are often countervailing interests that need to be considered. The result of these countervailing interests is the creation of a series of exceptions that justify the invasion of the interest of privacy in particular sets of circumstances.

---

3   s 12(4)(b) *Human Rights Act 1998*.
4   Other types of confidences are trade secrets, Government information, and artistic and literary confidences: *see* Francis Gurry. *Breach of Confidence*. Oxford: Clarendon Press; 1984.
5   *Source Informatics Ltd, Re: An Application for Judicial Review* [1999] EWCA Civ 3011, para. 34 per Simon Brown LJ.
6   *Wainwright v Home Office* [2003] UKHL 53, [2003] 4 All ER 969, paras. 31–32.

2.2.4   For the common law, the legal policy reason for upholding confidences is that it is in the public interest for confidences to be protected. This point is important when we begin to consider when a breach of the duty of confidentiality can be justified.

2.2.5   The question of confidentiality should be distinguished from the situation where the dissemination of untrue information results in harm. The latter is considered predominantly under rules of tort law, including the actions for defamation, libel and slander.[7]

2.3   EVOLUTION OF THE LAW

2.3.1   The main action available at common law is an action for **breach of confidence**. The Court has the power to intervene to prevent the disclosure of information which may come into one's possession where that information should not be divulged in all good conscience.

2.3.2   The power of the Court to intervene in these cases rests on an additional jurisdiction that it possesses, the **equitable jurisdiction**.[8] This jurisdiction operates to uphold the conscience of the recipient. It grants the Court the power to provide a remedy where a breach of a duty of confidence is threatened.[9]

2.3.3   The action for breach of confidence has been evolving over time to provide progressively more and more protection for the interest of privacy. The law of confidence has developed in the traditional way of the common law by a process of extending and developing existing principles. Whilst the Court can extend and develop existing causes of action if justice demands, it will not invent new causes of action to provide remedies where this is not appropriate.[10]

          'At times judges must, and do, legislate but . . . they do so only interstitially, and with molecular rather than molar motions.'[11,12]

2.3.4   Breach of confidence arises at the point of disclosure. Thus it is an indirect protection for the interest of privacy. It is possible to conceive of a new tort (*see* Section 1.3.11) that protects the interest of privacy

---

7   Other actions include negligent misstatement, deceit and the rule in *Wilkinson v Downton* [1897] 2 QB 57.
8   *Seager v Copydex Ltd.* [1967] 2 All ER 415, 435 per Lord Denning MR.
9   *Duchess of Argyll v Duke of Argyll* [1965] 1 All ER 611.
10   *Wainwright v Home Office* [2003] UKHL 53, [2003] 4 All ER 969, HL.
11   *Southern Pacific Co v Jensen* (1917) 244 US 205, 221 per Holmes J.
12   *Malone v Commissioner of Police of the Metropolis (No 2)* [1979] 2 All ER 620, 641.

from invasion. This new tort might have the properties of battery (*see* Section 3.3) but protect the interest of privacy rather than the interest in preventing others physically interfering with one's body. However, when offered the opportunity, this creative leap by intelligent design was eschewed by the House of Lords[13] through their approval of the reasoning in the decision of *Kaye v Robertson*.[14]

2.3.5   In *Kaye v Robertson* the famous 'Allo 'Allo actor Gordon Kaye was in Charing Cross Hospital having suffered a serious head injury in a car accident. Reporters from a tabloid newspaper entered his hospital room without permission, took photographs and asked Gordon Kaye questions despite the fact that he was unwell and unable to provide consent as a result of his head injury. An action seeking restraint of publication based upon a putative tort of privacy was unsuccessful on the basis that no such tort was known to English law. Breach of confidence was not raised as a cause of action and, therefore, was not considered by the Court.

2.3.6   This failure to create a general tort of privacy has arisen for several reasons:

(i)   the complexity of the task, which amounts to the amalgamation of a confluence of distinctly different legal principles (*see* Sections 2.2.1–2.2.4)

(ii)   because of a genuine reluctance by the judiciary to create new causes of action (*see* Section 2.3.3)

(iii)   in certain situations, because the more ponderous common law mechanism of developing law was not felt to be as suitable as an Act of Parliament for providing the necessary detailed exceptions to the broad principle of respect for confidence,[15] and

(iv)   the *Human Rights Act 1998* is felt to have the potential to fill many of the perceived gaps in the protection of the interest of privacy provided by the common law (*see* Section 2.5).[38]

---

13   *Wainwright v Home Office* [2003] UKHL 53, [2003] 4 All ER 969 per Ld Hoffman.
14   [1991] FSR 62 CA.
15   *Malone v Commissioner of Police of the Metropolis (No 2)* [1979] 2 All ER 620, 642, 647–8. This case lead to the *Interception of Communications Act 1985*.

2.4 BREACH OF CONFIDENCE

2.4.1 An action for breach of duty requires that three main ingredients must be present:[24,2]

(i) *Information that has the necessary quality of confidence.* Personal or intimate information will have this quality.[16] The information must be confidential, i.e. not already be in the public domain[17,18]

(ii) *The information was communicated in circumstances that import an obligation of confidence.*[24] The communication of information within the confines of a doctor–patient relationship is sufficient to import an obligation of confidentiality[18,19]

(iii) *The information must be used in an unauthorised manner* and some detriment must potentially result to the disclosing party from the use of the information.

2.4.2 Historically, such circumstances that imported an obligation of confidence arose from particular relationships that exist within society between individuals. These situations include:

(i) An express or implied term in a legal contract.[20] This may create a duty of confidentiality or may invoke a statutory obligation like those present in the *Official Secrets Act 1989*.

For example, in the new English consultant contract (2003), paragraph 8, schedule 12 of the terms and conditions of service imposes a contractual duty of confidentiality that extends not only to cover patients but also contractors and the confidential business of the employer organisation

(ii) Property rights can give rise to a common law duty of confidence in certain circumstances if they have been unlawfully invaded[21,22]

(iii) There may also be some aspect of the information that means that it amounts to a form of property (e.g. a patent or copyright). In this case the use and transfer of the information is limited because someone else owns those property rights. But the law of copyright differs from the rules about confidentiality in that the

---

16   *Barrymore (Michael) v News Group Newspapers Ltd* [1997] 24 FSR 600.

17   *Attorney General v Guardian Newspapers (No 2)* [1988] 3 All ER 545, 658 per Ld Goff.

18   *Observer and Guardian v the United Kingdom* [1991] ECHR 49.

19   *Hunter v Mann* [1974] 2 All ER 414, CA.

20   *Pollard v Photographic Co* (1888) 40 ChD 345.

21   *Prince Albert v Strange* (1849) 41 ER 1171.

22   *Saltman Engineering Co Ltd v Campbell Engineering Co Ltd* [1963] 3 All ER 413.

former can protect information in the public domain whilst the latter does not.

2.4.3   However the interest of privacy can be invaded in circumstances that where there is no pre-existing relationship between two people (e.g. the facts in *Kaye v Robertson, see* Section 2.3.4).[23]

2.4.4   In the *Spycatcher* case [1988],[24] Lord Goff gave the example of an obviously confidential document wafted out of a window by a fan and falling into the hands of a random passer-by on the street. After careful consideration he concluded that, in such a situation, the passer-by is bound by a duty of confidentiality despite the absence of any other relationship. He stated the general principle as being:

> 'that a duty of confidence arises when confidential information comes to the knowledge of a person (the confidant) in circumstances where he has notice, or is held to have agreed, that the information is confidential, with the effect that it would be just in all the circumstances that he should be precluded from disclosing the information to others.'[25]

2.4.5   Two other legal forces operate in addition to the common law to shape the landscape of the law of confidence:

(i)   The first is the *Human Rights Act 1998* which creates a right to respect for one's private and family life (Article 8). This right is counterbalanced by a right to freedom of expression (Article 10). This is considered in more detail below (*see* Section 2.5)

(ii)   The second are statutory provisions created by Parliament to prevent the misuse of information belonging to individuals and organisations in society in certain circumstances. A doctor's duty of confidence to his patient may be overridden by clear statutory language.

2.4.6   Three important examples of statutory limitations upon the medical professional's duty of confidence are:

(i)   *The Public Health (Control of Disease) Act 1984.*
This requires notification of a number of important notifiable diseases. This list (which has been subsequently supplemented[26])

---

23   For example, the unknown hearer in the phone tapping case of *Malone v Commissioner of Police of the Metropolis (No 2)* [1979] 2 All ER 620.
24   *Attorney General v Guardian Newspapers (No 2)* [1988] 3 All ER 545, HL.
25   *Attorney General v Guardian Newspapers (No 2)* [1988] 3 All ER 545, 657.
26   *Public Health (Infectious Diseases) Regulations 1988* SI 1988/546.

can be found on the Health Protection Agency website.[27] A small fee is payable for such notifications,[28] which need to be on a prescribed form[29]

(ii) *National Health Service (Venereal Diseases) Regulations 1974.*[30]
This protects the identity of people diagnosed with sexually transmitted diseases. It was considered in *X v Y*[31] (*see* Section 2.8.5). The exception permits communication of the identity to a medical practitioner (or people employed by a medical practitioner) for the purpose of treatment or prevention. The obligation is extended from GPs to cover NHS Trusts by virtue of a Direction to the NHS from the Secretary of State[32]

(iii) *The Data Protection Act 1998.*
This is an important piece of legal machinery that is explored further in Section 2.11.

2.4.7   In addition, Section 60 of the *Health and Social Care Act 2002* permits the Secretary of State to make regulations permitting the use of medical data without consent in order to help improve medical care or in the public interest. The use of data must be in accordance with the *Data Protection Act 1998* and not principally for the care given to an individual patient. Provision has been made under this section for the use of information in relation to neoplasia and communicable diseases.[33]

2.5   HUMAN RIGHTS AND CONFIDENTIALITY: ARTICLES 8 AND 10

2.5.1   The Court must decide any case before them in accordance with the rights set out in the *European Convention for the Protection of Human Rights and Fundamental Freedoms 1950* and included in Schedule 1 of the *Human Rights Act 1998* (the convention rights).[34]

2.5.2   In the context of the common law action for breach of confidence, these rights come into play once the information is disclosed with the

---

27   www.hpa.org.uk/infections/topics_az/noids/noidlist.htm.
28   s 12 *Public Health (Control of Disease) Act 1984.*
29   Schedule 2 *Public Health (Infectious Diseases) Regulations 1988* SI 1988/546.
30   SI 1974/29.
31   [1988] 2 All ER 648.
32   *NHS Trusts and Primary Care Trusts (Sexually Transmitted Diseases) Directions 2000* www.dh.gov.uk/en/Publicationsandstatistics/Publications/PublicationsLegislation/DH_4083027.
33   *Health Service (Control of Patient Information) Regulations 2002* SI 2002/1438.
34   ss 6(1)–(3) *Human Rights Act 1998.*

expectation of confidentiality.[35] In addition, Section 8 of the *Human Rights Act 1998* gives the Court power to provide a remedy where it is satisfied that convention rights are breached and no other remedy is available or sufficient.

2.5.3 Where there is a conflict between the common law and the Human Rights principles, the common law conclusion is overridden by the convention rights, e.g. the *Spycatcher* case.[24]

2.5.4 The two key rights that operate here are the Article 8: right to a private and family life, and a counterbalancing right to freedom of speech under Article 10. Neither right is absolute. Each is qualified by a set of competing interests that are set out in **Table 1** (*see* below).

TABLE 1 Comparision of interests qualifying the Article 8 and Article 10 rights.

Article 8: Right to a private and family life	Article 10: Right to freedom of speech
–	Territorial integrity
National security	National security
Public safety	Public safety
Prevention of crime or disorder	Prevention of disorder or crime
Protection of health or morals	Protection of health or morals
Protection of other people's rights and freedoms	Protection of the rights of others
Economic well-being of the country	–
–	Prevention of the disclosure of information received in confidence
–	Protection of the reputation or rights of others
–	Maintaining the authority and impartiality of the judiciary

2.5.5 In the simplest situation, the Article 10: right to freedom of speech can directly conflict with the Article 8: right to privacy. In more complex situations, the case may invoke the qualifying interests that restrict one or other of these rights.

2.5.6 **The Human Rights Approach:** This begins by asking if the Article 8 right is engaged, i.e. has the interest of privacy as protected by the right of privacy been invaded? If it has, the question then becomes whether the invasion can be justified. The invasion must be in accordance with

---

35 *Campbell v MGN Ltd* [2004] UKHL 22, [2004] 2 All ER 995, para. 138 per Baroness Hale.

the law and only to the extent necessary[36] in a democratic society. The extent of the lawful invasion must be justified by appealing to another conflicting right or interest. That other right or interest has to be legitimate (for examples, *see* **Table 1**). Further, the benefit gained from pursuing that other interest has to be proportionate to the harm caused by the invasion of the interest of privacy. In essence this is a balancing exercise.

2.5.7   For example, in one case the European Court of Human Rights held that the economic well-being of the country was an interest that justified the disclosure of medical notes.[37] In the next case, a breach of medical confidence by the Finnish Court was not justified.

Z v Finland [1997] ECHR 10

Z was HIV positive. Z was married to H who had initially been HIV negative.

H was alleged to have committed several indecent assaults. During the investigation the police discovered that H was HIV positive. Given that H was likely to have discovered that he had become HIV positive prior to at least some of the indecent assaults the police charged H with attempted manslaughter in additional to sexual offences.

The issue was when H came to know that he was HIV positive. To answer this question the police sought Z's medical records.

D was Z's doctor. D initially refused to surrender the records, but eventually gave evidence under Court order. The police subsequently seized Z's medical records, placing part of them into evidence.

Z was diagnosed to be HIV positive five months after marrying H whilst H was diagnosed HIV positive two years after the marriage. The Court inferred that H knew he was infected from symptoms he had which were present about 20 months after the marriage. On this basis, H was convicted of three counts of attempted manslaughter and one count of rape.

An abbreviated judgment was given. The full Court judgment which named Z and the case evidence would become available to the public, but this was not to be disclosed for 10 years. Finnish law permitted disclosure to be withheld for 30 years.

The press obtained the Helsinki Court of Appeal judgment containing the identity of Z, and her HIV status was obtained by the press who took up the case. They disclosed H's name and the fact that his wife was Finnish and HIV positive. Z sought a remedy in the European Court of Human Rights.

---

36   i.e. there must be a 'pressing social need'.
37   *MS v Sweden* [1997] ECHR 49.

Held: Z awarded 100,000 Finnish marks (approx £8,500 at that time) plus costs.

The ECHR regarded the protection of medical data as a fundamentally important expression of the Article 8 right to privacy. Z's interest of privacy was invaded by accessing the medical records and requiring evidence from D.

The use of the medical information for the investigation and trial was justified in the interests of preventing crime and protecting the interests of others.

Disclosing the identity of Z and the fact of her HIV status after the trial was not necessary in a democratic society. Disclosure of the identity of Z and her HIV status to the press through the judgment of the Helsinki Court of Appeal was unjustified.

Disclosure of the case records and full judgment only 10 years after the trial was a disproportionate infringement on Z's Article 8: right to privacy.

2.5.8   The English common law action of breach of confidence must now be seen in light of the convention rights.[38] Both protect the same underlying interest in privacy. The common law approach to seeking a justification for any breach of confidence is based on balancing the public interest in protecting confidences against the public interest in free speech.

2.5.9   By contrast the Article 8: right to privacy starts with a broad blanket of protection. Because of this the common law breach of confidence action has had to expand in scope, growing to cover a greater part of the interest in privacy. The common law approach is now infused by increasingly similar, but not yet identical, convention rights approach to the balancing of rights and interests.[39]

2.5.10   The result is that the convention rights and the common law justifications for invading the interest of privacy seem to be moving into alignment. For example, note in **Table 1** (*see* p. 12) how the Article 10 right is restricted by an interest in preventing the disclosure of information received in confidence. This dovetails with the common law structures.

---

38   *See*, for example, *Wainwright v Home Office* [2003] UKHL 53, para. 34.
39   *See*, for example, *Stone v South East Coast Strategic Health Authority* [2006] EWHC 1668.

2.6   ANONYMISED DATA

2.6.1   The use of anonymised data does not invade the interest of privacy where that interest in privacy rests on knowledge of the identity of the patient.

2.6.2   Patient confidentiality is distinct from patient autonomy (*see* Section 3.1). In the following case the Court of Appeal felt that patient autonomy is *not* the interest protected by the law of breach of confidence. It was on this basis that the Court of Appeal permitted the sale of anonymised patient data by pharmacists and GPs to a marketing company, despite the lack of patient consent to this use. Notice how the patient lacks any property rights in the information in this situation (*see* Sections 17.2–17.4).

Source Informatics Ltd, Re: An Application for Judicial Review [1999] EWCA Civ 3011, CA

Source Informatics Ltd S had sought to obtain the consent of pharmacists and general practitioners (GPs) to the obtaining of information about the prescribing practices of individual GPs in order to inform targeted marketing strategies. The data would be anonymised such that there would be no significant risk of patient identification. The consent of the patient to this disclosure would not be sought.

The Department of Health's policy operated to prevent the disclosure of this information.

S sought judicial review to declare that the policy of the Department of Health was unlawful.

Held: Use of anonymised data for this purpose was not unlawful.

The law of confidence protects the confider's (P) interest in privacy. The interest of patient autonomy is not protected by the law of confidentiality. P has no proprietary interest in the information.

Information is confidential if it can identify P. If the information is anonymised, the interest of privacy is not invaded. The consciences of the pharmacists would not be troubled by the disclosure of the anonymised information.

The use of anonymised data was not a misuse of information under a European data protection directive.[40] (This directive underlies the Data Protection Act 1998 (*see* Section 2.11), which was not then yet fully in force).[41]

2.6.3   The Achilles heel of this reasoning is the step of anonymising identifiable data for the purpose of subsequent disclosure to the company. The judgment implies that this was lawfully done in the circumstances. Such processing is now subject to the terms of the *Data Protection Act 1998* (*see* Section 2.11).

2.6.4   Note also that the concept of autonomy is a consideration within the protections provided by Article 8.[42] The decision in *Source Informatics* is grounded in a view of confidentiality based upon the original equitable doctrine (*see* Section 2.3). As we have seen, this base has been subsequently extended[35] such that the breach of confidence action should be interpreted in light of the convention rights, including Article 8.

2.6.5   It was important that the information was lawfully obtained and used by the pharmacists. This point distinguishes the case from $X v Y$[43] (*see* Section 2.8.5).

2.7   CONSENT

2.7.1   A disclosure of information protected by a duty of confidence can be undertaken with the express or implied consent of the person to whom the duty is owed.[44] The effect of consent is to modify the duty of confidence (*see* also para. 2.2.4). Therefore a duty of confidence owed to P cannot be used as a reason not to disclose to P.

---

40   Based upon Recital 26 of Directive 95/46/EC.
41   Fully in force 1 March 2000: *Data Protection Act 1998 (Commencement) Order 2000* SI 2000/183.
42   *Pretty v United Kingdom* [2002] ECHR 423, para. 61.
43   [1988] 2 All ER 648.
44   *Saltman Engineering Co Ltd v Campbell Engineering Co Ltd* [1948] 65 RPC 203, 213 per Lord Greene MR.

C v C [1946] 1 All ER 562

P and her husband H were in the process of divorce proceedings. P had been diagnosed as suffering from secondary syphilis. P asked her own doctor (D) to disclose to her and to H (who was also D's patient) the details of her condition. D refused on the grounds of confidentiality.

Held: The failure to disclose upon the request of the patient could not be justified by an appeal to the duty of confidence.

2.8 DISCLOSURE IN THE PUBLIC INTEREST

2.8.1 Unlike consent, which modifies the duty of confidentiality, the public interest overrides the duty of confidentiality.[45] Breach of confidence can be justified in the public interest where it is likely to relieve a serious risk to the health of the public. Note that the balancing process weighs the likelihood of the harm and the magnitude of the harm against the public interest in maintaining confidentiality.

2.8.2 In the next case, the issue was the disclosure in breach of confidence and whether this could be justified by virtue of the fact that there was a potential threat to the public. It is important to recognise that in this case there was no clearly identifiable potential victim. Contrast this case with the case where there is an identifiable potential victim (*see* Section 2.9).

W v Egdell [1990] 1 All ER 835, CA

W had killed five people and seriously wounded two others. He had been convicted of manslaughter on the grounds of diminished responsibility. Based on a diagnosis of schizophrenia he was remanded to Broadmoor secure hospital. After some time his doctor had completed a report suggesting that W might be suitable to enter a rehabilitation programme which had the potential for eventual release. The Secretary of State refused to accept this recommendation.

W sought to appeal this decision. W's solicitor engaged D by contract to provide an independent psychiatric report as part of this process. D assessed W as being a serious potential risk to the public *inter alia* because

---

45 *Source Informatics Ltd, Re: An Application for Judicial Review* [1999] EWCA Civ 3011 para. 53.

of an interest in firearms and explosives. W saw the report and withdrew the appeal application meaning that the Mental Health Tribunal would not receive D's report.

In breach of confidence D brought the report to the attention of the hospital medical director, who forwarded a copy to the Secretary of State.

W brought an action for breach of confidence, seeking to restrain disclosure and for damages for breach of confidence.

Held: There was a breach of the duty of confidence but that breach was justified by the public interest in preventing violence against the public.

The interests to be balanced are public interests. W's private interest in being released was not part of the balancing exercise.

There is a public interest in patients feeling able to make full and frank disclosure to their doctors. This interest was here outweighed by the public interest in protecting the public against possible violence.

2.8.3   Note that D did not have clinical responsibility for W. The relationship between D and W was based on a contract. D's justified breach of confidence, i.e. disclosing to the medical director, was narrow. A broader breach, for example to the press, may not have been as readily justifiable.[46]

2.8.4   Where the Court does not judge the threat to the public to be sufficient to outweigh the public interest in favour of maintaining confidentiality it will restrain the disclosure.[47] In such a case the Court may also restrain the disclosure of the identities of third parties where this might lead to the identification of the protected identity.[48]

2.8.5   In relation to free speech there is a difference between what the public is interested to know and what is in the public interest to disclose.[49]

---

46   For example, *Ashworth Security Hospital v MGN Limited* [2002] UKHL 29 where, based on preliminary facts, the hospital was able to discover the identity of a journalist's source of information. But in *Mersey Care NHS Trust v Ackroyd* [2007] EWCA Civ 101, the full facts of the case were considered and disclosure was not ordered.

47   *X v Y* [1988] 2 All ER 648.

48   *H (A Healthcare Worker) v Associated Newspapers Ltd* [2002] EWCA Civ 195.

49   *British Steel Corp v Granada Television Ltd* [1981] 1 All ER 417, 455 per Lord Wilberforce.

X v Y [1988] 2 All ER 648, QBD

The issue of HIV-positive professionals was the subject of widespread public debate. D1 and D2 were two GPs who were diagnosed HIV positive but were still practising. Through a breach of confidence a newspaper obtained the identities of the GPs, and sought to publish them, ostensibly in the public interest.

The evidence was that at that time there were only 11 known cases of transmission of HIV from patients to medical professionals, and none from medical professionals to patients. The Court accepted that the risk to the public was very low.

The *National Health Service (Venereal Diseases) Regulations 1974* (see Section 2.4.6) operated to preclude the hospital from disclosing the identity of the GPs.

Held: D1 and D2 were entitled to a permanent injunction restraining further disclosures.

The public interest in encouraging HIV-positive people to come forward for treatment and advice outweighed any public interest advanced by the newspaper as justification for disclosing the identities of the GPs.

2.9   PREVENTION OF DISORDER OR CRIME

2.9.1   Another situation where the public interest may justify a breach of confidence is where it is likely to prevent disorder or crime. In the Californian case of *Tarasoff v Regents of the University of California*[50] D became aware that their patient P intended to kill X who was an identifiable person. D warned the police, who briefly held P but subsequently released him. X was not warned of the threat to her. P went on to kill X. X's parents sought to establish that D had a duty to warn X of the risk to her life. The Court held (6:1) that there was an arguable case for failure to warn. Justice Clarke dissented on the basis that any disclosure would have caused a breach of medical confidence.

2.9.2   The case was in Californian law and was, in fact, subsequently settled out of court. If these facts arose here today, where there is an identifiable potential victim, a duty to warn the potential victim may exist. The necessary breach of confidence could arguably be justified on the basis that it would be likely to prevent disorder or crime. *See* also *W*

---

50   (1976) 17 Cal 3d 358.

v Egdell[51] (*see* Section 2.8.2). Where the victim remains unidentified then a duty to warn the third party was not found to exist.[52]

2.10 GMC GUIDANCE ON CONFIDENTIALITY: OVERVIEW

2.10.1 Appropriately, to accommodate professional practice, the GMC guidance on confidentiality[53] integrates a respect for the patient's autonomy in addition to the rules for protecting confidentiality. Thus, where disclosure is contemplated, it requires that the patient is informed of this prospect wherever practicable.

2.10.2 However, the guidance does permit disclosure where the patient withholds their consent to disclosure and there is a justification for disclosure other than the consent of the patient, e.g. a serious risk to the patient or others including situations of suspected abuse or neglect,[54] a legal obligation to disclose,[55] or disclosure in the context of legal proceedings.[56]

2.10.3 It also requires that consent for disclosure of patient identifiable information be sought from the patient before performing clinical tasks for a third party (*see*, for example, *W v Egdell*,[57] Section 2.8.2) or before disclosing such information for purposes such as research, epidemiology, financial audit or administration.[58] Disclosure of patient identifiable information is only permitted for clinical audit with the consent of the patient or where it is not possible to provide safe care without such disclosure.[59]

2.10.4 The guidance requires that patients should be made aware that their information will be shared within the healthcare team and with other care providers. One view is that this is because disclosure is intrinsic

---

51 [1990] 1 All ER 835.
52 *Palmer v Tees Health Authority* [1999] EWCA Civ 1533, CA.
53 GMC guidance. Confidentiality: Protecting and Providing Information. April 2004. www.gmc-uk.org/guidance/current/library/confidentiality.asp.
54 GMC guidance. Confidentiality: Protecting and Providing Information. April 2004. paras. 22–27, 29.
55 GMC guidance. Confidentiality: Protecting and Providing Information. April 2004. paras. 18 and 21.
56 GMC guidance. Confidentiality: Protecting and Providing Information. April 2004. paras. 19–20.
57 [1990] 1 All ER 835.
58 GMC guidance. Confidentiality: Protecting and Providing Information. April 2004. paras. 16–17.
59 GMC guidance. Confidentiality: Protecting and Providing Information. April 2004. paras. 13–15.

to their treatment. On this view such disclosure is based on an implicit consent to disclose because such information is necessary to deliver the treatment.[60]

2.10.5 For incompetent patients and in cases of emergency an appeal can be made to the Article 8 qualification of the protection of health or morals (*see* para. 2.5.4) to justify necessary disclosure.[61] However the GMC guidance requires involving advocates or carers with the agreement of the patient where possible.[62]

2.10.6 For competent patients whilst implied consent can permit disclosure it does not follow that a refusal to consent to disclosure based on the principle of patient autonomy gives a right to refuse disclosure if another justification can be found (*see*, for example, *Z v Finland*,[63] Section 2.5.7).[60] The GMC guidance also imposes an obligation to hold confidences, but the scope of this obligation 'will depend upon the circumstances'.[64] The Guidance once again lays great emphasis upon the principle of autonomy. But, as we have seen, the interest protected here is the interest in privacy.

2.10.7 It is unclear in law whether a duty of confidence is owed to the deceased. How the scope of any such duty of confidence owed to medical confidences after the death of a patient might be determined is illuminated by the following case. Here, medical confidences about the President of France were disclosed after his death. Note that French law maintains the obligation to hold medical confidences even after the patient dies.

Éditions Plon v France [2006] 42 EHRR 36, ECHR

D was a private physician to President Mitterrand of France. The President had advanced prostate cancer whilst in office. D sought to publish a book entitled *Le Grand Secret* ('The Big Secret') giving a detailed account of the

---

60 Kennedy I, Grubb A. *Medical Law*. 3rd ed. Butterworths; 2000: 1088–9.
61 Another case is *Woolgar v Chief Constable of Sussex Police* [1999] 3 All ER 604, CA where a police investigation revealed information about a nurse that was not sufficient to bring charges but was sufficient to justify disclosure to the nursing regulatory body (UKCC). An action to restrain the breach of confidence by the police failed. The disclosure was justified by appeal to the need to protect public safety, the protection of health or morals and the rights of others.
62 GMC guidance. Confidentiality: Protecting and Providing Information. April 2004; para. 28.
63 [1997] ECHR 10.
64 GMC guidance. Confidentiality: Protecting and Providing Information. April 2004; para. 30.

President's illness. It depicted the President as having misled the French people about the existence and duration of his illness.

The book was planned to be distributed about 10 days after the President's death. At this point in time the widow and children of the President successfully obtained a temporary injunction restraining publication.

Three months later the French Courts found D guilty of the French law criminal offence of breaching professional confidence. D received a sentence of four months suspended imprisonment.

Nine months later, a permanent injunction was granted against the further publication of the book despite the fact that the book had been widely published.

In the European Court of Human Rights (ECHR) the publishers, Éditions Plon, sought to lift the injunction on the basis of their Article 10: right to freedom of speech.

Held: Initial restraint of publication was justified but subsequent restraint of publication was not justified.

The distribution of the book was in breach of medical confidentiality.

The French Court could justify the initial restraint of publication on the grounds of the protection of the rights of the President and his family in the immediate aftermath of the President's death.

The subsequent permanent injunction restraining publication was not justified. It was granted over nine months after the President's death. By then the book had been published on the internet and 40 000 copies had been sold. This effectively destroyed the confidential quality of the information. In addition, the interests of the President and his family became less powerful as time passed.

2.10.8   The case was argued as a claim for the Article 10 right to override the French legal restriction upon disclosing medical confidences after death. The French Court of Appeal did not regard the right of privacy as continuing after death. However, the ECHR did not distinguish between the rights of the President and those of his heirs. It regarded the President's rights as vesting in his heirs. Thus it is unclear if the right of privacy can persist after death independently of the existence of living heirs. Subject to this caveat, the ECHR did recognise that the right of privacy was owed to the medical confidences of a deceased person. It was this right that permitted the temporary injunction lawfully restraining the freedom of the press. The scope of this right was determined by the balancing of interests approach.

2.10.9   Contrast this case with *X v Y*[65] (*see* Section 2.8.5) where there was also a disclosure of confidential information in bad faith, but, there, disclosure was restrained with a permanent injunction. The lack of a permanent injunction in *Éditions Plon v France* might seem a surprising result for an unlawful breach of medical confidence. However, the Court distinguished between the initial unlawful breach of medical confidence, which had been punished, and the right of the press to freedom of speech which was in issue. The initial balance favoured the rights of others, i.e. those of the President and his heirs because of their interest in privacy so soon after the President's death. But over time the weight of these interests waned. There is significant weight given to the freedom of the press.

2.10.10 The other main reason for the lack of a permanent injunction was that over time the book had entered the public domain. Importantly, the right of privacy requires that what is sought to be kept private has the quality of being private. This is because once information is in the public domain the law cannot restore privacy by putting the information genie back into the bottle. This point underlines the imperative to keep confidential patient information confidential.[39]

2.10.11 This need to retain a quality of privacy about the information mirrors the first criterion for a common law breach of confidence action (*see* Section 2.4.1). In the *Spycatcher* case a similar outcome resulted from the destruction of the confidential quality of the information by lawful publication of the book in Australia and the USA.[18]

2.10.12 Where the information is already in the public domain through a breach of confidence, the Court can offer money in the form of damages as partial recompense for the invasion of the interest of privacy where appropriate (for example, *Z v Finland*,[66] Section 2.8.5).

2.10.13 If the disclosure of medical information is already complete then breach in bad faith may justify invading the right of free expression in ways other than by restricting its exercise. In *Ashworth Security Hospital v MGN Limited*[67] the Daily Mirror newspaper published an article containing information from the medical records of the Moors murderer Ian Brady. The Hospital was successful in obtaining the opinion of the Court requiring that the newspaper disclose the identity

---

65   [1988] 2 All ER 648.
66   [1997] ECHR 10.
67   [2002] UKHL 29, HL.

of its source of the information. This invasion of the Press's right to free expression was justified because:

(i) it would be just and would deter further breaches if the person responsible for leaking the records was caught and punished

(ii) medical confidences should be protected in order to encourage patients to disclose information important for their health to medical professionals,[68] and

(iii) if medical confidences were not assured at Ashworth there may ultimately result a risk of crime or disorder.

2.10.14 In *Ashworth Security Hospital v MGN Limited*[69] the assumption was made that requiring MGN to reveal its source would reveal the source within the Hospital rather than the journalist providing the story. *Mersey Care NHS Trust v Ackroyd*[70] was a subsequent action against the journalist to obtain the identity of the source within the Hospital but the disclosure of the identity of the Hospital source was not ordered. This decision rested in part on the change in circumstances that had occurred over the time between the 2 trials.

2.10.15 Within the NHS, one way to disclose iniquity with a degree of legal protection is to use the provisions of the *Public Interest Disclosure Act 1998*. Briefly, this provides statutory protection for employment where disclosure reveals unlawful activity, miscarriages of justice, risks to health and safety or the environment, or that such matters have been concealed. Such disclosure must be made in good faith *inter alia* to the employer or other responsible person or to a legal advisor. There must not be the prospect of personal gain, and the discloser must reasonably believe that the information is substantially true and that it is reasonable for them to make the disclosure.[71]

2.11 DATA PROTECTION ACT 1998 AND ACCESS TO MEDICAL RECORDS

2.11.1 The *Data Protection Act 1998* is a piece of legislative machinery which gives effect in English law to a European data protection directive.[72]

---

68   *Z v Finland* [1998] 25 EHRR 371, para. 94–5.
69   [2002] UKHL 29, HL.
70   [2007] EWCA Civ 101; preceeded by *Ackroyd v Mersey Care NHS Trust* [2003] EWCA Civ 663.
71   ss 43A-L *Employment Rights Act 1996* and HSC 1999/198.
72   EC Directive 95/46/EC .

It is broad and relatively detailed. Here we will only deal with a few of the aspects most relevant to this discussion.

2.11.2 Unlike breach of confidence and the convention rights, the *Data Protection Act 1998* operates to regulate information in the form of data. It indirectly promotes both the interest of privacy and the interest of self-determination. The *Data Protection Act 1998* adds to the existing framework. It ensures this by importing the entire common law of confidentiality into its structure.

2.11.3 The way the *Data Protection Act 1998* achieves this goal is by requiring that any processing of data must be lawfully conducted.[73] Thus the regulatory framework it provides in relation to how data can be acquired, accessed, handled and stored incorporates the pre-existing legal framework. The facts of *Source Informatics*[74] (*see* Section 2.6.2) provide an example of how these structures operate together.

2.11.4 **Data** is widely defined and includes any form of information that is stored in an organised accessible record, including electronic or non-electronic health records.[75,76]

2.11.5 **Personal data** is data from which the identity of a living individual (the data subject) can be ascertained, including situations where another piece of information that is likely to be available to the person processing the data can be used to identify the data subject.

2.11.6 **Sensitive personal data** includes information that relates to the data subjects' physical or mental health, including their sexual life.[77]

2.11.7 The individual or organisation that determines the purpose for which the data is to be used (i.e. 'processed') is the **data controller**. For data controllers, personal data must not be processed without registration.[78] Within the NHS, data controllers are often an NHS body.

2.11.8 Any person who processes personal information on behalf of the data controller is a **data processor**. Processing again is widely defined to include storing, using, altering and erasing the information, but also includes disclosure of the information.[73,39]

---

73   Schedule 2, para. 1 *Data Protection Act 1998*.
74   [1999] EWCA Civ 3011.
75   s 1(1) *Data Protection Act 1998*.
76   s 68(1)(a) *Data Protection Act 1998*.
77   s 2 *Data Protection Act 1998*.
78   s 17 *Data Protection Act 1998*.

2.11.9 Processing of personal data must be done in accordance with the **data protection principles**:[16] processing must be done fairly and lawfully; it must be done for at least one specified lawful purpose; processing other than for the specified purpose(s) is not permitted; the data must be accurate, relevant and both adequate and not excessive in light of the specified purpose(s); the data must be kept up to date and not for longer than is necessary to achieve the specified purpose(s); the data must be protected from accidental loss, damage or misuse; the data should not be exported to a country outside the European Economic Area unless adequate protections are available there; and the processing of the data must be done in accordance with the rights of the data subject.[79]

2.11.10 The Act grants the data subject a **right of access** to the information stored as personal data. This also includes information held about the source of the data, a description of the specified purposes for which the data is being or to be processed, and identification of anyone to whom the data might be disclosed. The right is exercisable by a request in writing.[80] The payment of a fee may be required.[81]

2.11.11 This right provides the data subject a means of accessing their own medical records. Note that records compiled before 1 November 1991 are accessible under this provision, unlike the situation when the relevant provisions of the *Access to Medical Records Act 1990* were in force.

2.11.12 Where another person can be identified by this information due regard must be had to any duty of confidentiality owed to the other individual.[79] Disclosure is not restricted on this basis if this other person is a heath professional involved in the care of the data subject.[82]

2.11.13 In the case of medical records, the right of access is subject to an exception where such access might cause serious harm to the physical or mental health of the data subject or other person.[83] The decision to disclose information on this ground must be made by, or after consultation with, a health professional currently or most recently

---

79 Schedule 1 *Data Protection Act 1998*.
80 s 7 *Data Protection Act 1998*.
81 The current maximum fee is £50 for health records. Regulation 6 *Data Protection (Subject Access) (Fees and Miscellaneous Provisions) Regulations 2000* SI 2000/191 amended by *Data Protection (Subject Access) (Fees and Miscellaneous Provisions) (Amendment) Regulations 2001* SI 2001/3223.
82 s 7(4)(c) *Data Protection Act 1998* inserted by Regulation 8 *Data Protection (Subject Access Modification) (Health) Order 2000* SI 2000/413.
83 Regulation 5 *Data Protection (Subject Access Modification) (Health) Order 2000* SI 2000/413.

involved in the care of the data subject or another qualified health professional.[84]

2.11.14 Another important exemption is where the request is made on behalf of a child by someone with parental responsibility. Disclosure can be refused if, when the information was provided or obtained, the expectation of the data subject was that it would not be disclosed to the person applying for the information.[82]

2.11.15 A further right is the **right to rectify inaccurate personal data**. This requires an application to the Court who must be satisfied that the information sought to be rectified is inaccurate.[85]

2.11.16 The data subject also had a **right to require the data controller to stop (or not start) processing personal data for any purpose or in any manner that is likely to cause them substantial unwarranted damage or distress**.[86] The processing can be justified in such cases on several grounds, including that the processing is necessary to protect the vital interests of the data subject and that the processing is necessary to fulfil a legal obligation.

2.11.17 Data processing must be done in accordance with the data protection principles (*see* Section 2.11.9). The Department of Health Guidance on records management[87] suggests that the processing will be fair if the patient was not misled into giving the information, and they had basic information about the specified purpose for processing the information and who will be processing the information.

2.11.18 For personal data the processing must be justified.[88] The grounds for such justification include: consent of the data subject; in order to meet a legal obligation other than one imposed by a contract; the processing is necessary to protect the vital interests of the data subject; or the processing is necessary for legitimate purposes pursued by the data controller. For legitimate medical care, if we interpret legitimate purposes to include protection of the subject's vital interests and the protection of health and morals, we can leap this hurdle even in the absence of formal consent.[89]

---

84 Regulation 6 *Data Protection (Subject Access Modification) (Health) Order 2000* SI 2000/413.
85 s 14 *Data Protection Act 1998*.
86 s 10 (1) *Data Protection Act 1998*.
87 www.dh.gov.uk/en/Policyandguidance/Organisationpolicy/Recordsmanagement/ DH_4000489 (accessed: 14/09/2007 17: 20).
88 s 4(3) *Data Protection Act 1998*.
89 Schedule 2 *Data Protection Act 1998*.

2.11.19　Processing of sensitive personal data (such as medical records) must be additionally justified.[90] The available justifications include: explicit consent of the data subject (note that implied consent is insufficient); the processing is necessary for medical purposes and is undertaken by a health professional or person bound by an equivalent duty of confidence; or, if consent cannot be given or reasonably obtained, processing is necessary to protect the vital interests of the data subject or other persons. Once again, for use in legitimate medical care these grounds can almost always be met.

2.11.20　Personal data processed only for research purposes (including statistical purposes) are exempt from the right of access provision. The data must not be used in relation to decisions relating to particular individuals or processed such that substantial damage or distress is caused to any data subject, and the results must not disclose the identity of the data subjects.[91]

2.11.21　Research findings can be kept indefinitely.[90] The information must still be processed lawfully and fairly (*see* Sections 2.11.2 and 2.11.17).

2.11.22　Data held on the Human Fertilisation and Embryology Authority's register of information is exempted from the provisions of the *Data Protection Act 1998*.[92] Disclosure is regulated by the *Human Fertilisation and Embryology Act 1990*.[93]

2.11.23　Information contained in medical notes is exempt from access by the data subject under the provisions of the *Freedom of Information Act 2000* because it is personal information[94] and because it is accessible to the data subject by other means.[95]

2.11.24　There are three other situations where access to medical records might be required. The first is in the context of **legal proceedings**. Where legal proceedings are contemplated but not yet in process, an application can be made to the Court requesting access to documents including medical records that might be relevant.[96] In such cases the party from whom the documents are sought does not need to be contemplated as a party to any proceedings.[97] Once proceedings

---

90　s 4(4) *Data Protection Act 1998*.
91　ss 33(3),(4) *Data Protection Act 1998*.
92　Part 1 *Data Protection (Miscellaneous Subject Access Exemptions) Order 2000* SI 2000/419.
93　s 33 *Human Fertilisation and Embryology Act 1990*.
94　s 40(1) *Freedom of Information Act 2000*.
95　s 21 *Freedom of Information Act 2000*.
96　s 33 *Supreme Court Act 1981*.
97　s 34 *Supreme Court Act 1981*.

are in process, relevant records can be obtained thorough litigation disclosure rules (for example, the disclosure requirements of the pre-action protocol).[98]

2.11.25 The second is access under the *Access to Health Records Act 1990* where the patient (data subject) has died. The need for this provision arises from the fact that the protection of the *Data Protection Act 1998* for personal data does not extend after death of the data subject.[99] Here an application to the holder of the patient's health records can be (i) the executors or personal representatives of a person who has died, or (ii) any person who might have a claim arising out of the patient's death. Note that an application to the Court is not required.

2.11.26 However, the value of such an application is limited by the fact that it can be refused by the record holder on a number of grounds:

(i) the patient had refused disclosure by a written statement present in the medical notes

(ii) the information was provided by the patient in the expectation that it would not be disclosed to the applicant

(iii) the information is a result of an examination or investigation that the patient consented to undertake in the expectation that it would not be disclosed in this context

(iv) where the holder of the record believes it might cause serious harm to the mental or physical health of any person (note the subjectivity of this test), or

(v) the information may identify a third party who is not either a healthcare professional involved in the care of the patient, or has not consented to their identity being revealed.

2.11.27 The third is access under the *Access to Medical Reports Act 1988* to a medical report made for employment or insurance purposes by a doctor who is or has been responsible for the care of the patient. The point here is that the medical report is not created in connection with the care of the individual.[100] This provision does overlap the *Data Protection Act 1998* right which might be used to obtain access in many of these cases.

---

98   Rule 31 *Civil Procedure Rules.*
99   s 1(1) *Data Protection Act 1998.*
100 s 68(2) *Data Protection Act 1998.*

2.11.28 Under the *Access to Medical Reports Act 1988* the party seeking the report (the applicant) must notify and obtain the consent of the patient to applying for the report.[101] When the patient gives their consent they may require that they have access to the report before it is released to the applicant.

2.11.29 The doctor must permit the patient access to the report upon the request of the patient, prior to supplying the report or for six months afterwards.[102] Two exceptions to this principle are essentially the same as those in Section 2.11.26 (4) and (5) above – i.e. serious harm and identification of a third party. A third exception is dissimilar: where such disclosure would reveal the intentions of the doctor in relation to the patient.

2.11.30 If accessing the report prior to supply to the applicant then the patient must consent to the supply of the report to the applicant. Before giving their consent, the patient may request in writing that the doctor change any part of the report that the patient regards as being incorrect or misleading. If the doctor does not accept such a request then the patient may refuse consent to disclosure or, if the patient desires, the doctor must attach a statement of the patient's views to the report as they relate to such unamended parts.[103]

2.12 CONCLUSION

2.12.1 The basic interest protected is the interest of privacy. It is protected by the common law equitable doctrine of breach of confidence. The introduction of the Article 8: right to a private and family life has added an extension to the protection of the interest of privacy. Further protections are provided by statute, in particular the *Data Protection Act 1998*.

2.12.2 The protection for the interest of privacy is not absolute. Other interests, both of the individual and society, can and do weight more heavily in certain situations.

---

101 s 3 *Access to Medical Reports Act 1988.*
102 ss 4, 6 *Access to Medical Reports Act 1988.*
103 s 5 *Access to Medical Reports Act 1988.*

3 Consent: general

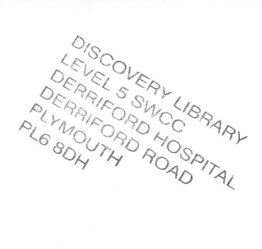

3.1 THE ESSENCE OF CONSENT

3.1.1   Consent can be thought of as either:

(i)   the competent expression of freely given, comprehending acquiescence to what is proposed, or

(ii) a legal justification for the invasion of an individual person's right to be free from physical interference.

3.1.2   These two concepts lie at the heart of the idea of consent, with one or other often taking a more prominent role depending upon the situation. Much of the apparent complexity of this area of law results from the underlying presence of these two concepts.

3.1.3   From a personal standpoint there is great value in having the power to shape your own life through the decisions you make yourself. The ethical principle of respect for autonomy states that it is morally good to respect the choices made by others. The prime goal of medicine is to promote the welfare of the patient. In medical practice respect for patient autonomy powerfully contributes to this prime goal. This is because a patient is more likely to gain from a treatment that they willingly accept.[1]

3.1.4   The legal expression of personal autonomy has a positive and a negative aspect, both resting upon the interest of self-determination (*see* Section 3.1.8).

3.1.5   The negative aspect of personal autonomy is a privilege[2] which has the effect of negating the duties owed by medical professionals to the patient. This privilege rests on the interest of self-determination.

---

1   *See*, also, *Re: W (a minor) (medical treatment)* [1992] 4 All ER 627, 632 per Ld Donaldson on the purpose of consent.

2   Hohfeld, WN. In: Cook WW, eds. *Fundamental legal conceptions as applied in judicial reasoning.* New Haven, CT: Yale University Press; 1919 (reprint 1964)).

3.1.6　The positive aspect of the legal expression of personal autonomy can be regarded as a power[3] to alter legal relationships in pursuit of the interest of self-determination.

3.1.7　Over time, the interest of self-determination is emerging as a greater and greater force within the legal structure. To accommodate this emergence, common law could not simply create causes of action based on this interest (*see* Section 2.3.3). Therefore, it looked to existing legal structures and sought to develop them to better accommodate the interest in self-determination. One major legal tool exploited was the action for battery (*see* Section 3.3) which protects the interest in being free from unjustified physical interference. Consent is one defence to this action.

3.1.8　In 1914, Cardozo J famously connected consent as a defence to battery and the interest in self-determination:

> '. . . Every human being of adult years and sound mind has a right to determine what shall be done with his own body; and a surgeon who performs an operation without his patient's consent commits an assault, for which he is liable in damages.'[4]

This connection has been developed in the subsequent case law.

3.1.9　Self-determination has two aspects:

(i) a freedom (or privilege) not be prevented from pursuing your goals; and

(ii) a claim to have others act to promote your goals.

The former materialises as a right to be free from unjustified physical interference and imposes negative obligations upon others. It is a shield to protect oneself from the actions of others. The latter claims to impose obligations upon others to do positive things to advance your goals. It is a sword to drive the actions of others. Confusion can arise because the term 'right to self-determination' has been used in relation to both these distinct aspects. Here, the right to self-determination implies the privilege not the claim right[5] unless stated otherwise.

3　Hohfeld, WN, op. cit.
4　Per Cardozo J in *Schloendorff v Society NY Hospital* (1914) 211 N.Y. 125 approved in 129 above per Goff Ld.
5　Hohfeld, WN, op. cit.

3.1.10   The interest in self-determination and the interest in being free from unjustified physical interference are not coterminous, and rarely this can give rise to apparent injustice (*see* Section 6.2.7).

3.1.11   It is important to be clear that consent is a shield not a sword. This means that consent cannot enlarge the duties owed by a medical professional to their patient.

Burke v GMC [2005] EWCA Civ 1003, CA

P was a 45-year-old man suffering from spino-cerebellar ataxia, resulting in progressive disability and a poor prognosis. The condition did not affect his cognitive function. The evidence was that P would remain competent until the final stages of the disease.

In those final stages P would initially loose the ability to communicate but would retain his sentience. He would soon thereafter lapse into a coma. During those final stages artificial nutrition and hydration (ANH) would no longer be capable of prolonging his life.

P desired that ANH should be provided even after he became incompetent. P's concern was that doctors would determine for him whether or not ANH would be provided.

He challenged, inter alia, paragraphs 32 and 81 of the GMC Guidance published in 2002 entitled *Withholding and Withdrawing Life-prolonging Treatment: Good Practice and Decision Making*. Paragraph 32 declared that the responsibility of withholding or withdrawing life-prolonging treatment was that of the consultant or general practitioner in charge of a patient's care. This decision should be made taking into account the views of the patient and those close to the patient.

Paragraph 81 empowered the responsible doctor to withdraw life-prolonging ANH where it might cause suffering or be too burdensome in relation to the possible benefits.

Held: It is unlawful for a doctor to withdraw life-prolonging ANH from a competent patient where this withdrawal is contrary to the wishes of the patient.

Whilst not strictly necessary to disposing of the case the Court approved the following GMC statement:

'If . . . [the patient] refuses all of the treatment options offered to him and instead informs the doctor that he wants a form of treatment which the doctor has not offered him, the doctor will, no doubt, discuss that form of treatment with him . . . but if the doctor concludes that this treatment is not clinically indicated he is not required (i.e. he is under no legal obligation) to provide it to the patient although he should offer to arrange a second opinion.'

3.1.12 Whilst this is an admirably clear and mercifully brief decision when compared to the first judgment, the difficulty is that it begs the definition of 'clinically indicated'. It can be argued whether this term means that the treatment promotes the welfare of the patient, or the best interest of the patient, or simply accords with the modified *Bolam* test (*see* Section 10.4).

3.1.13 Where the patient is not competent, then the interest in self-determination is not pursuable and the actions of those responsible for the patient should be driven by the best interests of the patient. This situation is now additionally subject to the provisions of the *Mental Capacity Act 2005* (*see* Section 4.8).

3.2 THE LIMITS OF CONSENT

3.2.1 The State has an interest in our physical welfare. This public interest can, in extreme situations, limit the autonomous power of a competent person to consent to physical injury.[6] Therefore, consent is not a defence to murder[7] (*see* Sections 19.6.8–19.6.9). Nor is consent a defence to a charge of actual bodily harm.[8] In the next case a consensual desire for sexual gratification was insufficient to make consent effective as a defence to a charge of actual bodily harm.[9]

R v Brown [1993] 2 All ER 75, HL.

Over a 10-year period a group of sado-masochistic male homosexuals willingly took part in acts of violence for sexual gratification. These acts included the insertion of sterilised fish hooks into the urethra, genital torture with sandpaper and genital piercing. The acts of violence occurred in private and no lasting physical injury was suffered. None of the appellants had any medical qualifications.

---

6   *R v Coney* (1882) 8 QBD 534, 553 per Hawkins J.
7   *R v Cox* (1992) 12 BMLR 38.
8   *R v Brown* [1993] 2 All ER 75.
9   *R v Donovan* [1934] 2 KB 498; although note *R v Wilson* [1996] TLR March 5.

The acts were videoed. These videos were not sold for profit but were distributed amongst the group to use for their private personal pleasure.

The events were not reported to the police. The police obtained copies of the tapes and used them to prosecute members of the group for the crimes of assault occasioning actual bodily harm[10] and unlawful wounding.[11,12]

At first instance Rant J ruled that conviction was possible without the need to prove absence of consent on the part of the victim of the violence. Members of the group appealed, contending that the presence of consent precluded conviction. The Court of Appeal dismissed the appeals. The group made a further appeal against conviction to the House of Lords.

Held (3:2): Conviction upheld.

3.2.2   In *R v Brown*[13] the consent of the participants to the actual bodily harm was not a valid defence. By analogy an invasive surgical procedure amounts to the intentional infliction of actual bodily harm upon the patient. This leads us to question the basis upon which a surgeon performing an invasive surgical procedure can justify the invasion of the patient's physical integrity.

3.2.3   The fact that consent to a surgical procedure amounts to a defence for the surgeon's invasion of the patient's physical integrity must rest on more than a profound respect for patient autonomy alone. One could argue that, in general, the lawfulness of surgery is based upon its potentially therapeutic effect. However, the fact that it is lawful to remove a donated organ (for example, a kidney) for the benefit of another person challenges this view.[14]

3.2.4   What makes invasive surgical procedures lawful is a legal policy decision that it is in the public interest for operations performed by a skilled surgeon to be legally permissible.[15,16,17] The key idea is that

---

10   s 47 *Offences Against the Person Act 1861*.

11   s 20 *Offences Against the Person Act 1861*.

12   To constitute a wound for the purposes of the section the whole skin must be broken and not merely the epidermis: *J J C (a minor) v Eisenhower [1983] 3 All ER 230*, Crim QBD Goff LJ, Mann J – air gun pellet causing bruising below left eye and blood in front of part of the left eye held not to be wounding.

13   *R v Brown* [1993] 2 All ER 75.

14   *Attorney-General's Reference (No 6 of 1980)* [1981] 2 All ER 1057.

15   *R v Brown* [1993] 2 All ER 75.

16   *Attorney-General's Reference (No 6 of 1980)* [1981] 2 All ER 1057.

17   Law Commission. Consent in the Criminal Law (Consultation Paper) [1995] EWLC C139, para. 8.31–2.

medicine overall does not harm patients but, in fact, operates to promote the health of the public.[18]

3.2.5 Rational as it might seem at first, if this was the only justification necessary for invasive surgical procedures then consent would not be required. But, despite generally promoting the public interest, a surgical procedure also invades the patient's interest of being free from unjustified physical interference. Therefore, consent or other legal justification is needed to justify the invasion of this latter interest – even for skilled surgeons.

3.2.6 Within this framework it seems unlikely that the intentional infliction of serious physical harm, or even death, for the benefit of another would be lawful.[19] So it seems likely that the donation of a heart from one person to another (outside a domino transplant scenario – *see* para. 18.10.15) would not be permitted.[19] However, this has yet to be tested in court.

3.2.7 An additional legal structure that impacts upon this area of law is the *Mental Capacity Act 2005* (*see* Section 4.8). It operates in relation to incompetent adults. Within this framework, consent can operate either as an expression of the patient's choice (through advance decisions or the choices made by a patient-appointed proxy decision-maker) or as a legal justification for an intervention (via statutory consent which can be given by the Court under the *Mental Capacity Act 2005*).

3.2.8 In relation to questions of the adequacy of information provided about the proposed medical procedure the Courts do not use the tort of battery, instead they look to the tort of negligence (*see* Section 6.4).

3.2.9 Fortunately, medical professionals almost always[20,21] lack sufficient intention to harm, which precludes criminal sanctions from applying.

3.3 BATTERY

3.3.1 Battery is the intentional and direct application of force upon another without lawful justification. Assault is an action by another that

---

18 *Airedale NHS Trust v Bland* [1993] 1 All ER 821, 886–7 per Mustill LJ.
19 Law Commission. Consent in the Criminal Law (Consultation Paper) [1995] EWLC C139 (15 January 1995).
20 Murder: *R v Cox* [1968] 1 All ER 386; Dr Harold Shipman: http://news.bbc.co.uk/1/hi/uk/3391871.stm.
21 Manslaughter: *R v Adomako* [1994] 3 All ER 79.

reasonably[22] causes the victim to apprehend the immediate infliction of a battery.

3.3.2 The legal rule is that *in the absence of a lawful justification, any touching of another's body may be actionable in law*. This protection extends not only against physical injury but against any form of physical molestation.[23]

3.3.3 One exception to this rule against touching is the physical contact that is generally acceptable in the ordinary conduct of everyday life.[24] However, medical treatment, even treatment for minor ailments, does not fall within this exception.[25] Treatment without the consent of the patient may lead to a legal action and the award of damages, or even criminal sanctions, against the medical professional concerned.[26]

3.3.4 The consent of a competent patient to the touching necessary to deliver medical care amounts to a lawful justification for the purposes of battery. An eminent judge, Lord Donaldson likened consent to a legal 'flak-jacket' for the medical practitioner.[27]

3.3.5 There are many other interests that conflict with the interest to be free from unjustified physical interference, so there are many ways to legally justify invasion of this interest. For example, the police possess statutory powers of arrest that ground in the societal interest to uphold the rule of law.[28]

3.3.6 Assault and/or battery can result in an action for damages in the civil courts. If committed intentionally or recklessly,[29] assault and battery are also criminal offences[30] and, if tried in the magistrates courts, the punishments in these cases include a fine and up to six months imprisonment.[31] In practice, such criminal charges are rarely brought against medical professionals.

3.3.7 It is important to recognise that the basic premise of the rules surrounding battery and consent have nothing to do with how well or badly a medical procedure is performed, or even whether the patient

---

22 'Reasonable' has a special meaning in law – *see* para. 10.1.7.
23 Robins JA in *Malette v Shulman* [1990] 67 DLR (4th) 321, Ont CA.
24 *Wilson v Pringle* [1986] 2 All ER 440, CA.
25 *F v West Berkshire Health Authority* [1989] 2 All ER 545, 563 per Lord Goff.
26 *F v West Berkshire Health Authority* [1989] 2 All ER 545, 563 per Lord Goff.
27 *Re:W (a minor) (medical treatment)* [1992] 4 All ER 627.
28 For example, s 1 *Police and Criminal Evidence Act 1984*; s 41 *Terrorism Act 2000*.
29 Probably *Cunningham* recklessness: *R v Spratt* [1991] 2 All ER 210.
30 *Offences Against the Person Act 1861*.
31 s 39 *Criminal Justice Act 1988*.

benefited from the procedure or not. Whether a procedure was well or badly performed is addressed by the courts through the tort of negligence (*see* Sections 8–11).

3.3.8   Thus, even a procedure that is expertly performed and benefits the patient can result in a successful action for battery if it is done without the consent of the patient or other lawful justification.

Mohr v Williams [1905] 104 NW 12, Minnesota

An ENT surgeon (D) obtained the consent of P for a procedure on the right ear. Whilst P was under general anaesthetic D discovered a more serious problem with the left ear. D proceeded to perform a successful procedure on the left ear relieving the problem.

Held: D had not been negligent but damages were awarded against D for operating without consent.

3.3.9   Similarly, if a medical professional obtains consent to one procedure and performs another they may be liable in battery.[32]

Devi v West Midlands RHA [1980] C.L.Y. 687

P was a 29-year-old married woman with four children. She consented to a minor operation on her uterus. Her religious beliefs forbade contraception or sterilisation. At surgery her uterus was found to be ruptured. Without consent the surgeon (D) performed a hysterectomy to preclude the risk of uterine rupture during any future pregnancy.

Held: D was liable in battery because there was lack of consent to the operation performed.

3.4   COMPETENCE AND CONSENT

3.4.1   The question of competence is issue-specific, i.e. it relates to the question the patient must answer.[33]

---

32   *Williamson v East London and City HA* (1998) BMLR 85 – no consent to additional procedure during explant breast prosthesis.
33   *Masterman-Lister v Brutton & Co* [2002] EWCA Civ 1889.

3.4.2   A *competent patient* is a patient who is legally capable of giving their consent. Once they have established that they have legal competence they can refuse consent to treatment for 'any reason, rational or irrational, or for no reason at all'[34] even if they lose their life or suffer significant harm as a result of this choice (*see* Sections 4.5 and 5.4).

3.4.3   An *incompetent patient* is a patient who is not able to give consent (for example, young children, some mentally-disabled patients and unconscious patients). For these patients, consent can be given by others (for example, those with parental responsibility, lasting powers of attorney or the Court). In this context consent is not clearly an expression of patient autonomy; rather, it amounts to a legal justification for the touching that is medically justified. As such, it is constrained by the best interests of the patient (*see* Sections 4.6–4.14 and 5.5).

3.5   EVIDENCE OF CONSENT

3.5.1   For competent patients consent is a state of mind.[35] In order to justify the medical touching it becomes necessary to establish that the patient had the state of mind called consent at the relevant point in time. Because a Court cannot read minds it must look to the evidence to determine what the state of mind of the patient was at the time of the medical treatment. This means that a medical professional can rely on evidence that consent was present at the time of the medical treatment against a *post hoc* counter-claim that consent had not been given.

3.5.2   A contemporaneously signed written consent form is powerful evidence of the existence of consent at the time of the medical contact. But a signed piece of paper purporting to be evidence of the state of mind of consent would not be sufficient if, for example, no explanation of the proposed treatment had in fact been given.[36] Demonstration of the existence of consent does not need to be in any particular form.[37] For example, consent may verbal or even implied from the circumstances. The next case demonstrates both of these principles in action.

---

34   *Re: MB* (1997) 8 Med LR 217, CA per Butler-Sloss LJ.

35   *Sidaway v Bethlem Royal Hospital Governors* [1985] 1 All ER 643, 657 per Diplock Lord.

36   *See* Bristow J in *Chatterton v Gerson* [1981] 1 All ER 257, 265.

37   *Re: T (adult: refusal of treatment)* [1992] 4 All ER 649, 653 per Lord Donaldson MR.

O'Brien v Cunard SS Company (1891) 28 N.E. 266 (Mass Sup Jud Ct).
Knowlton J

P was on a boat carrying emigrants to America. D was a doctor on the
boat. While on the boat P offered her arm to receive a vaccination from D
and D vaccinated her. P subsequently sued D for battery claiming that she
had not consented to the vaccination.

Held: No battery.

D successfully relied on the offered arm as objective evidence of
consent.

3.5.3　　This argument applies to situations where consent is the competent
expression of freely given, comprehending acquiescence to what is
proposed. Where consent is a legal justification for the invasion of the
individual's right to be free from physical interference the existence
of that justification must be established. For example, the power of a
parent in relation to a child to consent on behalf of the child rests, in
part, upon establishing that the parent does indeed possess parental
responsibility in relation to that child (*see* Section 5).

4 Consent: adults

4.1 THE TEST FOR COMPETENCE: ADULTS

4.1.1 In order to establish that a competent decision has been made, three core elements must be present:

> (i) the patient must have legal capacity to consent (*see* paras. 4.1.2–4.1.9)
>
> (ii) the consent must given voluntarily (*see* Section 4.2), and
>
> (iii) the consent must be informed (*see* Section 6)

4.1.2 **Capacity:** A person is presumed to have capacity unless it can be established that they lack capacity.[1] Therefore, it rests on a person asserting a lack of capacity to demonstrate that lack of capacity on a balance of probabilities. Medical practitioners must, therefore, be in a position to assess the capacity of patients prior to diagnosis or treatment decisions in almost all cases.

4.1.3 In general, a person lacks capacity if,[2] because of some impairment or disturbance in the functioning of their brain or mind,[3] they cannot:

> (i) understand the information relevant to the decision
>
> (ii) retain that information[4]

---

1 s 1(2) *Mental Capacity Act 2005*.
2 *Re: MB* (1997) 8 Med LR 217. Note that ss 2, 3 *Mental Capacity Act 2005* essentially codifies this case law.
3 s 1(2) *Mental Health Act 2007* amends the definition of 'mental disorder' within the *Mental Health 1983* to: 'any disorder or disability of the mind' which may impact upon this definition.
4 The information needs to be retained long enough for P to make the decision: para. 4.20 *Mental Capacity Act 2005 Code of Practice*. Department for Constitutional Affairs. www.dca.gov.uk/legal-policy/mental-capacity/ (accessed 31.3.2007).

(iii) use or weigh that information as part of the process of making the decision,[5,6] or

(iv) communicate their decision.[7,8]

4.1.4   If a person lacks capacity in relation to a particular decision they are incompetent in relation to that decision. It does not follow necessarily that they lack competence in relation to all choices they might have to make. The degree of competence required to make a particular decision increases with the gravity of the decision.[9] Thus, a person may not be competent in relation to a decision involving the refusal of life-preserving treatment, but may be competent to select which flavour of ice-cream they would prefer after dinner. All possible practical steps must have been taken to enable capacity before a person can be judged to be incompetent[10] and, if incompetent, a person should still be involved in the decision-making process as far as practicable.[11]

4.1.5   It is only necessary to have capacity at the time of making the decision. Thus, the fact that the information is not subsequently retained does not mean that the person was incompetent at the time of making the decision.[12] For an example of a situation where P was unable to understand the relevant information necessary to make a competent decision see the next case.

State of Tennessee v Northern (1978) 563 SW 2d 197 (Tenn Ct App)

P had gangrene of both feet. She refused consent to surgery. P refused to recognise her own feet as 'dead black shrivelled rotting and stinking'; she also refused to consider the eventuality of death.

Held: Not competent to refuse consent.

---

5   *R v Collins and Ashworth Hospital Authority* ex parte *Brady* (2001) 58 BMLR 173 – Moors murderer Ian Brady inter alia found incompetent by virtue of his personality disorder to refuse force feeding whilst on hunger strike. Could also be force fed under s 63 *Mental Health Act 1983* as a medical treatment for his mental disorder.
6   *Re: MB* (1997) 8 Med LR 217, CA per Butler-Sloss LJ.
7   *Re: MB* (1997) 8 Med LR 217, CA per Butler-Sloss LJ.
8   See Section 4.4.1 for an explanation of this rule.
9   *NHS Trust v T (adult patient: refusal of medical treatment)* [2005] 1 All ER 387, 402 per Charles J.
10   s 1(3) *Mental Capacity Act 2005.*
11   s 4(4) *Mental Capacity Act 2005.*
12   s 3(3) *Mental Capacity Act 2005.*

4.1.6   There is an additional requirement present in case law *to believe the information*.[13,14] This is necessary in addition to taking in the information and using it as part of the decision-making process (*see* Section 4.1.3).

4.1.7   Even where the information is believed and understood, the decision may still be incompetent. This can arise where the understanding is grounded in a misperception of reality attributable to an impairment or dysfunction of brain or mind.[3] In *NHS Trust v T (adult patient: refusal of medical treatment)* (below), the impairment of mind was the borderline *personality* disorder. This impairment of mind lead to the persisting misperception by P that her blood was evil. Her understanding of the situation was based on this misperception. This flawed basis of her understanding undermined the validity of her refusal to consent to further blood transfusions.

NHS Trust v T (adult patient: refusal of medical treatment) [2005] 1 All ER 387, Fam

P was a 37-year-old woman who suffered from a persisting borderline personality disorder. She harmed herself intermittently by cutting, resulting in severe anaemia that required blood transfusions.

P executed an advance directive whereby she refused consent to further blood transfusions even if they were necessary to save her life. She declared that she believed that her 'blood was evil'.

P was admitted suffering from severe anaemia. The Hospital applied for an order that blood transfusion was lawful.

At first instance an order was granted permitting blood transfusion.

The Hospital then applied for an interim declaration that blood transfusion would be lawful to preserve P's life or avert immediate risk of serious injury to her health. This was on the basis that this would be likely to be a recurring problem.

Held: Interim declaration granted.

P lacked capacity and this state was likely to persist. To guard against a change of circumstances, P's solicitors and the Official Solicitor should be notified if P was readmitted or a decision was made to transfuse P.

The Court had power under para. 25(1)(b) of the *Civil Procedure Rules* to grant an interim declaration.

---

13   *Re: C (adult: refusal of medical treatment)* [1994] 1 All ER 819.
14   This is not a separate criterion within the *Mental Capacity Act 2005*. It is possible that it will be subsumed within the need to understand the information relevant to the decision.

4.1.8   However the mere fact of a disturbance or impairment in the functioning of someone's mind is not sufficient to make them incompetent. The level of irrationality that is necessary to make a decision incompetent is high. It must be 'so outrageous in its defiance of logic or of accepted moral standards that no sensible person who had applied his mind to the question to be decided could have arrived at it'.[15] Thus the mere fact that there is delusional thinking may not actually affect the ability of the patient to believe or understand the information relevant to making the material decision.

Re: C (adult: refusal of medical treatment) [1994] 1 All ER 819[16]

P was a 68-year-old male suffering from chronic paranoid schizophrenia. He suffered grandiose delusions including the belief that he was a doctor with an international medical career during which he had not lost a single patient.

P was suffering from a gangrenous right foot. P was seen by a surgeon who offered P amputation of the afflicted foot estimating a 15% chance of survival without surgery and a 15% mortality with surgery.

P refused amputation.

Held: The presumption in favour of P's competence had not been displaced on the evidence. P was competent to refuse treatment.

4.1.9   Whether a particular person has capacity in the context of a particular decision is a matter of fact to be considered in light of the available evidence. This reasoning was applied in the next case.

Re: JT (adult: refusal of medial treatment) [1998] 1 FLR 48

P was a 25-year-old female who had a learning disability associated with severe behavioural disturbance. P was detained under Section 3 of the *Mental Health Act 1983*.

P required haemodialysis for renal failure. P refused this, resisting the treatment on 11 occasions. The options of renal transplant and continuous ambulatory peritoneal dialysis (CAPD) were not suitable.

---

15   *NHS Trust v T (adult patient: refusal of medical treatment)* [2005] 1 All ER 387, 402 per Collins J. Compare this to Wednesbury unreasonableness: *Associated Provincial Picture Houses Ltd v Wednesbury Corporation* [1947] 2 All ER 680 and para. 1.3.11.

16   *See,* also, *Lane v Candura* (1978) 376 NE 2d 1232 (Mass App Ct).

The medical evidence was that she was competent to refuse the treatment. She understood she would die if she was not treated. The NHS Trust sought a declaration that withholding treatment was not unlawful.

Held: Patient was competent to refuse dialysis.

Patient satisfied the *Re: C*[17] test. The Court rejected the argument that dialysis was treatment for P's mental health.

4.2   CONSENT MUST BE VOLUNTARY

4.2.1   Even if the patient has capacity to make the decision, external influences must not operate to overbear the independence of the decision. Factors that might affect this independence are the strength of will of the patient and the relationship of the person who may be exercising the undue influence.[18]

Re: T (adult: refusal of medical treatment) [1992] 4 All ER 649, CA

P was about 20 years old. She had been brought up as a Jehovah's Witness but was not herself a Jehovah's Witness. P's mother was a fervent Jehovah's Witness who had separated from P's father when P was three years old.

P suffered a car accident when she was 34 weeks pregnant, and subsequently became unwell with a respiratory infection. P's mother spent some time alone with P, after which P signed a form refusing consent to blood transfusion.

P went into labour and required caesarean section. The child was stillborn. P was unconscious. She had deteriorated post partum, suffering from a lung abscess, and was transferred to the intensive care unit. The medical evidence was that she required a blood transfusion.

P's father sought a declaration from the Court that the transfusion was not unlawful. P's mother did not give evidence.

Held: P could lawfully receive the blood transfusion.

P's refusal to consent to the transfusion did not, on the evidence, extend to refusing life-saving treatment. If it did, it was vitiated by the undue influence[19] brought to bear by P's mother upon P's decision.

---

17   *Re: C (adult: refusal of medical treatment)* [1994] 1 All ER 819.
18   *Re: T (adult: refusal of medical treatment)* [1992] 4 All ER 649, 661 per Ld Donaldson MR.
19   'sapped her will and destroyed her volition' *Re: T (adult: refusal of medical treatment)* [1992] 4 All ER 649, 656 per Ward J cited by Ld Donaldson MR.

4.2.2   On the other side of the line was *U v Centre for Reproductive Medicine*[20] (*see* Section 15.2.13) where a challenge to vitiate a withdrawal of consent on the basis of undue influence was unsuccessful.

4.3   FLUCTUATING COMPETENCE

4.3.1   It is possible to have general competence but still be incompetent to face a particular decision. There are situations where competence can fluctuate.

Re: MB (1997) 8 Med LR 217, CA

P was a 23-year-old generally competent woman who was 40 weeks pregnant. P required caesarean section because of threatened breech birth. P had a needle phobia. She consented to the caesarean section, but once she was in the anaesthetic room she refused consent whenever she was approached by someone carrying a needle. She returned to consenting once the needle was taken away.

Held: P's needle phobia was such that it temporarily rendered her incompetent. Therefore the anaesthetist could administer anaesthetic without her consent as this was in her best interests.

4.3.2   Note that in this case it was ordered that reasonable force could be used if necessary.

4.4   CONSENT AND THE ABILITY TO COMMUNICATE

4.4.1   A person who cannot communicate their decision lacks capacity to consent to the proposed treatment (*see* Section 4.1.3). From the perspective of those making medical decisions about the patient, including the Court, the patient is incompetent. This is the position taken by case law[21] and the *Mental Capacity Act 2005*.[22]

4.4.2   This outcome flows from practical reality. In theory if we use consent as a tool to protect personal autonomy then the views of any conscious, sentient person should be respected. However, if that person is unable

---

20   [2002] EWCA Civ 565.
21   *Burke v GMC* [2005] EWCA Civ 1003, CA.
22   s 3(d) *Mental Capacity Act 2005*.

to communicate their wishes then in practical reality we cannot know the content of that person's desires. Our attempt to respect patient autonomy is thus defeated.

4.4.3   Where we use consent as a legal justification we lack evidence upon which to conclude either that the person consents to the proposed treatment or that they do not consent to the proposed treatment. Therefore, in practical reality, if the patient lacks the capacity to communicate a mental state then there is no way that relevant decision-making by others can be affected by that patient's mental state.

4.4.4   The *Mental Capacity Act 2005* does, however, impose a requirement that all practical steps have been taken to ensure that the patient can make a decision.[23] This could relate purely to the decision-making process and not apply to the process of communication. It is submitted, however, that this provision does require that reasonable steps to enable communication should be taken.[24]

4.5   REFUSAL OF CONSENT COMPETENT: ADULTS

4.5.1   Consent operates powerfully to protect the choices of the individual. The power of consent is such that it operates even if a decision to refuse consent made by a competent person results in that person suffering avoidable injury or even death.[25]

4.5.2   In *Re: B (adult: refusal of medical treatment)*[26] a 41-year-old woman suffered tetraplegia after bleeding into a cervical cavernoma. She was ventilator-dependent and made a competent request that the ventilation be removed. The Court held that the patient had the right to refuse the life-saving treatment.[27,28] A similar result arose in

---

23   s 1(3) *Mental Capacity Act 2005*.

24   *See* s 3(d) *Mental Capacity Act 2005*, where inability to make decisions is defined.

25   For example, *see Malette v Shulman*, which was a competent refusal to life-saving blood transfusion by a Jehovah's Witness.

26   [2002] EWHC 429 (Fam), [2002] 2 All ER 449, CA.

27   *Bouvia v Superior Court* (1986) 225 Cal Rptr 297 (Cal CA) was a Californian case about a 28-year-old with cerebral palsy refusing NG feeding. The competent refusal was valid, although the patient subsequently accepted alternative treatment.

28   In the Canadian case of *Nancy B v Hôtel-Dieu de Québec* (1992) 86 DLR (4th) 385, P was a competent 25-year-old woman who suffered complete paralysis from Guillain-Barré syndrome. She had all her mental faculties but could not breathe and depended for continued life on a ventilator. Her refusal of treatment was also upheld.

the tragic case of *Re: AK (Medical treatment: consent)*[29] *(see* Section 4.10.1).

4.5.3   But the power of consent is even greater than this. A maternal refusal of consent can operate to override the obligations owed by society and medical professionals to a fetus. This is so even where the life of the fetus and indeed the mother is at risk. This is because the Court gives high regard to a pregnant mother's right to refuse offered treatment.

St George's Healthcare NHS Trust v S [1998] 3 All ER 673, CA

P was a 31-year-old veterinary nurse who was 36 weeks pregnant.

She was suffering from severe pre-eclampsia which placed both her life and the life of the fetus at risk. P was competent and understood the risks but refused consent to caesarean section because she wanted to allow nature to 'take its course'.

P was detained for assessment under Section 2 of the *Mental Health Act 1983*.

At a first instance hearing, where P was not represented, the Court permitted caesarean section without her consent. The operation was performed and a healthy baby girl was delivered. No specific treatment for mental disorder or mental illness was prescribed.

P appealed against the first instance decision.

Held: Detention under the Mental Health Act was not justified on the facts. The caesarean section had been a trespass to the person (battery) and therefore unlawful.[30]

4.5.4   Note that in *St George's Healthcare NHS Trust v S (see* Section 4.5.3) P was not represented at the first instance hearing which was held in circumstances of some urgency. Guidelines issued in that case included

---

29   [2001] 1 FLR 129.

30   A series of earlier cases were considered but a clear new direction was set with *St George's Healthcare NHS Trust v S* [1998] 3 All ER 673 continuing along the road marked out by *Re: MB* (1997) 8 Med LR 217, CA. The earlier series of cases were: *Re: S (adult: refusal of medical treatment)* [1992] 4 All ER 671, *Norfolk and Norwich Healthcare NHS Trust v W* [1996] 2 FLR 613. The decision in *Re: S (Adult: refusal of medical treatment)* [1992] 4 All ER 671, where an emergency caesarean section was declared lawful despite the existence of a competent refusal of consent, was doubted in St *George's Healthcare NHS Trust v S* [1998] 3 All ER 673. It was also doubted in *Re: MB* (1997) 8 Med LR 217 and is unlikely to be good law.

the important point that in future cases P should be represented for hearings held in similar situations even where urgency was present.[31]

4.6 INCOMPETENT ADULTS

4.6.1 The legal rules surrounding decisions relating to the medical care of incompetent adults have been radically revised by the provisions of the *Mental Capacity Act 2005*. We will first consider the case law (common law) rules that evolved prior to the introduction of the *Mental Capacity Act 2005*, since these will still operate in situations where the *Mental Capacity Act 2005* does not apply. We will then consider the new legislative framework.

4.6.2 The *Mental Capacity Act 2005* overrides the common law rules where it operates (*see* Section 1.3.8). It is important to realise this, and to understand that where the Act does not operate the common law rules still apply.

4.7 INCOMPETENT ADULTS: CASE LAW

4.7.1 At common law the Court does not possess power to consent to a treatment on behalf of an incompetent adult. The power of the Court to consent to treatment on behalf of an incompetent adult did exist prior to 1 November 1960. It subsisted as a *parens patriae* jurisdiction (i.e. father of the people) vested in the Court in relation to incompetent adults akin to the jurisdiction currently available to the Court in relation to children (*see* Section 5.2.5).

4.7.2 On 1 November 1960 the *Mental Health Act 1959* (now replaced by the *Mental Health Act 1983*, as amended) came into force, and at the same time the residual powers of the Court over persons of unsound mind were revoked.[32] The effect was to remove the power of the Court to consent to medical treatment on behalf of an incompetent adult.[33,34]

4.7.3 Given this, the deep common law principle which most commonly justifies the invasion of the interest that the incompetent patient has

---

31 If necessary, this could be by the Official Solicitor as *amicus curiae*.
32 By warrant under the sign manual dated 10 April 1956.
33 *F v West Berkshire Health Authority* [1989] 2 All ER 545, HL.
34 There are first instance *obiter dicta* that suggest that the present power of the Court is equivalent to the old *parens patriae* jurisdiction: *Re: SA (vulnerable adult with capacity: marriage)* [2005] EWHC 2942 (Fam) para. 12 per Munby J.

in being free from unjustified physical interference is the principle of **necessity**.[35]

4.7.4 **Emergency** is a justification but does not cover all the situations where touching is done during the delivery of medical care.[36] For example, emergency cannot justify the nursing care of a chronically confused patient. The touching is necessary to discharge the duty of care. Emergency is simply one aspect of the deeper principle of necessity which operates where there is immediate risk of avoidable mental or physical harm.

4.7.5 It is important to note that invading the interest of personal liberty on the basis of the principle of necessity in patients with a mental disorder has been found to be in breach of the Article 5 right to liberty enshrined in the *Human Rights Act 1998*.[37] The changes introduced by the *Mental Health Act 2007* are designed to cure this gap in English law by creating an appropriate legislative framework. Space limitations preclude further exploration of this point here.

4.7.6 Other justifications for invading the interest of being free from unjustified physical interference do exist. They protect other interests that are socially desirable such as the interest in preventing the spread of communicable diseases,[38] and a societal interest in assisting people in need of care and attention and preventing such people causing serious nuisance.[39] We will not consider these further.

4.7.7 The **principle of necessity** operates where, in the absence of any other justification, a medical professional would be in breach of their duty of care if they did not touch the patient (*see* also Section 19.8). The duty of care and the justification of necessity are coterminous where the duty of care demands physical contact with the patient.

4.7.8 The scope of the principle of necessity and the scope of the duty of care are circumscribed by the test of best interests. This is because:

(i) The goal of medicine is to promote the welfare of the patient

(ii) A duty of care is owed by the medical professional to their patient (*see* Chapters 8–10). This duty requires that the medical

---

35   *F v West Berkshire Health Authority* [1989] 2 All ER 545, HL.
36   *F v West Berkshire Health Authority* [1989] 2 All ER 545, HL.
37   *HL v United Kingdom* (2004) 40 EHRR 761; *R v Bournewood Community and Mental Health NHS Trust ex p L* [1998] 3 All ER 289, HL.
38   ss 37–40 *Public Health (Control of Disease) Act 1984*.
39   s 47 *National Assistance Act 1947*.

professional should act (or not act if appropriate) to promote the welfare of the patient

(iii) In relation to an incompetent patient, the test to determine where the welfare of the patient lies is the best interests test (*see* Section 7).

4.7.9　This point makes it possible to see how, by working within the ambit circumscribed by the best interests test, one can develop a different framework of rights and duties in relation to incompetent adults. This new framework need not rely on the medical professional duty of care alone, it could rest upon the best interests of the patient.

4.7.10　Such a new framework can successfully interlock with the underlying case-based framework where needed. The mechanics of the new statutory framework deriving from the *Mental Capacity Act 2005* are based on this approach. Conceptually it is predicated on two ideas:

(i) Respect for the ethical principle of patient autonomy is a powerful way to promote a patient's welfare

(ii) Better decisions can be made in relation to a patient's best interests where such decision-making does not rest solely upon the medical duty of care.

4.8　INCOMPETENT ADULTS: MENTAL CAPACITY ACT 2005

4.8.1　The *Mental Capacity Act 2005* aims to enable the individual patient's choices wherever possible, and it also increases the protection of the best interests of the patient in other situations. It promotes patient choices through the use of **advance decisions** or patient-selected proxy decision-makers. Patient-selected proxy decision-makers will receive powers in relation to decisions surrounding the incompetent patient's personal welfare by virtue of a new legal device, the **lasting power of attorney (LPA)**.

4.8.2　Incompetent patients are particularly vulnerable when there is no one who can be appropriately consulted about where their best interests might lie. This is most acute when there are important choices to be made. When there are only responsible medical professionals or paid carers to consult and the incompetent patient lacks an advance decision or a proxy decision-maker, then the best interests of the patient are to be safeguarded by a new body of **independent mental** capacity advocates (IMCAs).[40] Their role is to function as an independent advocate for the incompetent patient.

4.8.3   **Research subjects** also gain additional protections. These protections apply to subjects involved in protocols involving intrusive research where consent to touching would ordinarily be required.[41] Clinical trials subject to the clinical trial regulations are excluded since they are covered by other legislation.

4.8.4   There are requirements in relation to approval of the research[42] and consultation with carers,[43] and additional safeguards including that interests of the patient must be assumed to outweigh those of science and society.[44]

4.8.5   In addition, a criminal offence of ill treatment or neglect[45] has been created by the *Mental Capacity Act 2005*.[46]

4.8.6   Importantly, this new structure does not weaken the underlying duties owed by medical professionals to their patients. It aims to operate by empowering patient-led decision-making and increasing the protection given to the best interests of vulnerable incompetent adults. To support this new structure there is a new judicial service, the **Court of Protection** that will, over time, develop expertise in the supervision of the affairs, both medical and financial, of incompetent adults.[47]

4.8.7   The Court of Protection will have broad powers to make decisions on behalf of incompetent adults.[48] It will have power to grant or refuse consent on behalf of the incompetent patient.[49] This statutory power to grant consent will return to the Court some of the power it had previously lost (*see* Section 4.7.1). Notice that this statutory consent is, in fact, a form of legal justification permitting the medical touching. It is not, except perhaps indirectly, an expression of patient autonomy akin to the common law consent that operates in relation to competent adults. In this sense, statutory consent is, in fact, a legal protective

---

40   s 37 *Mental Capacity Act 2005*.
41   s 30(1),(2) *Mental Capacity Act 2005*.
42   s 31 *Mental Capacity Act 2005*.
43   s 32 *Mental Capacity Act 2005*.
44   s 33 *Mental Capacity Act 2005*.
45   s 44 Mental Capacity Act 2005.
46   The *Mental Capacity Act 2005* (Commencement No.1) Order 2006 SI 2006/2814.
47   ss 45–56 *Mental Capacity Act 2005*.
48   s 16 *Mental Capacity Act 2005*.
49   s 17(1)(d) *Mental Capacity Act 2005*.

device that will function to promote the best interests of incompetent adults.

4.8.8   The Court of Protection will also have the power to appoint **court deputies** (who can be empowered to make decisions on behalf of the patient),[50] and **court visitors**,[51] whose role is to advise the Court and the Public Guardian.

4.8.9   The **Public Guardian** supports the Court of Protection. Its functions will include holding a register of lasting powers of attorney, registering and supervising court deputies, directing Court of Protection visitors, and dealing with complaints about how donees of LPAs exercise their powers.[52] We will not consider the details of the Court of Protection or the Public Guardian further here.

4.8.10   In addition to the rules contained in the Act itself, there is guidance contained in a **code of practice**[53] which should be complied with in the absence of there being good reasons to the contrary.[54] The *Mental Capacity Act 2005* does not cover patients who have mental disorders that require treatment. These patients continued treated under the *Mental Health Act 1983* as amended.[55]

4.9   ADVANCE DIRECTIVES AND ADVANCE DECISIONS

4.9.1   In essence, an advance directive or advance decision is a separation in time of a competent decision and the implementation of that decision. The fact that the decision is made at a different time does not grant any less nor any more power to the patient at the time of implementation than the patient would have had if they had made a contemporaneous competent decision.[56,57,58]

4.9.2   Whilst an advance directive or advance decision does not increase the force of competent decision, what it does do is to allow a competent decision made at one point in time be projected to a point in time when the decision-maker is incompetent.

---

50   s 16 *Mental Capacity Act 2005*.
51   s 61 *Mental Capacity Act 2005*.
52   s 58 *Mental Capacity Act 2005*.
53   Code of Practice, *Mental Capacity Act 2005*. www.publicguardian.gov.uk.
54   *R v Mersey Care NHS Trust* ex parte *Munjaz* [2005] UKHL 58.
55   s 28 *Mental Capacity Act 2005*.
56   *Burke v GMC* [2005] EWCA Civ 1003, CA.
57   s 26(1) *Mental Capacity Act 2005*.
58   para. 9.1 Code of Practice, *Mental Capacity Act 2005*. www.publicguardian.gov.uk.

4.9.3   If a patient becomes incompetent then the general rule at common law is that they should be treated in accordance with their best interests. However, the best interests test does not operate in relation to competent adults.[56] Where the advance directive or advance decision has the force of a competent decision projected through time it can supersede the best interests test. Granting such decisions this degree of force rests upon the acceptance of the validity of a claim based upon the interest of self-determination where the decision is made prior to becoming incompetent.

4.10   ADVANCE DIRECTIVES: CASE LAW

4.10.1   Where a valid advance directive exists that covers the actual circumstances that arise, then the expressed wishes of the patient should be respected.[59] Notice that it is in this situation that the best interests test conflicts most powerfully with the wishes of the patient. In the next case, P wished to have care withdrawn once he was 'locked in'. The difficult question is what would be the result of the best interests test for someone with locked-in syndrome if they had not made an advance decision?[60]

Re: AK (Medical treatment: consent) [2001] 1 FLR 129

P was 19 years old and had a 2½ year history of progressive motor neurone disease. P was ventilator-dependent. He had a vestigial amount of movement left in one eyelid with which he used to communicate. It was likely that, in time, this too would be lost. P desired that ventilation should be discontinued two weeks after he lost the last remnants of voluntary movement.

D sought a declaration from the Court that withdrawal of ventilation would be lawful.

Held: Given the express wishes of P, and subject to the continuing expression of those wishes, it would be unlawful to continue invasive ventilation two weeks after P completely lost voluntary movement.

4.10.2   The fact of separation in time between the decision and the implementation creates uncertainties. People's views change over time and

---

59   *St George's Healthcare NHS Trust v S* [1998] 3 All ER 673, CA.
60   *See*, for example, *Auckland Area Health Board v A-G* [1993] 1 NZLR 235.

people's actual reactions to certain situations may differ from those they might have anticipated. Therefore, where the advance directive refuses life-sustaining treatment the Court will need to be certain that the patient had made a fully informed and competent decision and intended the refusal to have effect in the circumstances that in fact arise.[61]

4.10.3 The burden of proving the validity and applicability falls to the person seeking to apply the advance directive. The impact of the principle of the sanctity of life is that where there is doubt it is to be resolved in favour of life.[61]

HE v A Hospital NHS Trust [2003] EWHC 1017, Fam[62]

P was a 24-year-old woman with congenital heart disease. Her father was a Muslim whilst her mother had become a Jehovah's Witness. P had signed an advance directive refusing transfusion of blood or blood products. This advance directive purported to operate even should P become incompetent.

P subsequently developed septic shock, secondary to acute bacterial endocarditis. On admission, she declared to her brother in the presence of a witness that she did not want to die. After being in hospital for two days P deteriorated and needed to be sedated and presently remained unconscious. In accordance with the advance directive P received non-blood volume replacement, vasopressors, erythropoietin and iron, together with haemofiltration.

Despite this, P deteriorated with an increasing level of plasma lactate and signs of peripheral necrosis. The medical evidence was that P required urgent blood transfusion to stand any chance of continued survival.

P's mother and brother remained adamant that no transfusion should be undertaken. P's father applied urgently to the Court for an order permitting blood transfusion. P's father gave evidence that:

(i) P had rejected her faith as a Jehovah's Witness and reverted back to the Muslim faith when recently becoming betrothed to a Turkish man

(ii) The advance directive pre-dated the betrothal

(iii) P had not mentioned the advance directive during her admission to hospital.

---

61 *See*, also, *W Healthcare NHS Trust v KH* [2004] EWCA Civ 1324.
62 *Ex tempore.*

Held: Blood transfusion could be lawfully given.

The burden of proving the existence, validity and applicability of an advance directive is upon those seeking to rely upon the advance directive.

The standard of proof is the balance of probabilities. The more serious the issues at stake the greater the weight of evidence is required to reach this standard of proof.

Advance directives could be made orally or in writing. Therefore, they could be revoked orally or in writing.

An irrevocable advance directive is a fettering of autonomy, a contradiction of terms. Any term purporting to make an advance directive irrevocable or only conditionally revocable is void on public policy grounds.[63]

There is an assumption that the advance directive has not been revoked. This assumption was rebutted by the evidence.

It was the fact of the betrothal and the reversion to Islam that carried evidential weight rather than the expression of the desire not to die. The latter could be expressed by a Jehovah's Witness who continued to adhere to their faith.

4.10.4   In *Re: T (adult: refusal of medical treatment)*[64] (*see* Section 4.2.1) the Court concluded that the evidence was that the advance directive did not extend to cover life-saving treatment.[65] Contrast this with *Burke v GMC*[66] (*see* Section 3.1.10) where the advance directive did cover life-saving treatment, but the treatment requested was such that it may not have fallen within the doctors' duty of care because it may have been of futile value (*see* Section 19.9) and thus could not be enforced. From this case note that futility trumps autonomy. *A fortiori* a demand for a futile treatment in the future cannot be enforced.

4.11   ADVANCE DECISIONS: MENTAL CAPACITY ACT 2005

4.11.1   An advance decision is distinct from an advance directive. The advance decision is a creature created by the *Mental Capacity Act 2005*. It is must be a decision made by an adult (18 years or older) who has capacity. It relates to a particular treatment that may arise in circumstances that the person making the advance decision specifies.

---

63   *HE v A Hospital NHS Trust* [2003] EWHC 1017, para. 39.
64   [1992] 4 All ER 649.
65   *Re: T (Adult: Refusal of Treatment)* [1992] 4 All ER 649, 660 per Ld Donaldson.
66   [2005] EWCA Civ 1003.

They can specify whether or not the treatment should be carried out or continued.[67] The fact that the advance decision is expressed in lay terms does not detract from its validity.[68]

4.11.2 The Code of Practice to the *Mental Capacity Act 2005* states that a person cannot use an advance decision to refuse comfort care including warmth, shelter, actions to keep a person clean, and the offer of food and drink by mouth.[69]

4.11.3 The Code of Practice also explains that advance decisions are about refusal of treatments. It is only in these situations that the duty of care owed by the medical professional is altered by the advance decision.[70] This result arises because there is a duty of care to carry out treatments that are in the best interests of incompetent patients. Offering an advance decision accepting such treatment does not alter the duty to deliver such treatments.

4.11.4 There is no duty to deliver treatments that are not clinically indicated.[71] The presence of consent to a treatment that is not clinically indicated does not create a duty to deliver the treatment (*see* Section 3.1.10). Only where there is a duty to deliver a treatment and consent is withheld does the refusal of consent change the duty of care from one requiring delivery of the treatment to one requiring the treatment to be withheld.

4.11.5 Life-sustaining treatment is treatment that a healthcare professional providing treatment regards as necessary to sustain life.[72] For treatments other than life-sustaining treatments, advance decisions can be made without writing, and altered or withdrawn without writing, provided the person making the advance decision has capacity and the alteration does not apply to any life-sustaining treatment.[73]

4.11.6 For treatments that are potentially life-sustaining the advance decision must be in writing, witnessed, and signed directly or indirectly by the adult making the advance decision. The advance decision must verify that it applies even when the adult's life is at risk.[74] Provided the adult has capacity, such decisions can be wholly withdrawn verbally. They

---

67 s 24 *Mental Capacity Act 2005.*
68 s 24(2) *Mental Capacity Act 2005.*
69 para. 9.28 Code of Practice *Mental Capacity Act 2005*. www.publicguardian.gov.uk
70 para. 9.5 Code of Practice *Mental Capacity Act 2005*. www.publicguardian.gov.uk
71 *Burke v GMC* [2005] EWCA Civ 1003, CA.
72 s 4(10) *Mental Capacity Act 2005.*
73 s 24 *Mental Capacity Act 2005.*
74 s 25(5) *Mental Capacity Act 2005.*

can also be altered or partially withdrawn verbally unless the resulting advance decision still applies to life-sustaining treatment, in which case the written formalities apply.[73]

4.11.7 An advance decision is not valid in relation to a particular treatment in prospect if:

(i) the adult has capacity to make the decision at the relevant time[75]

(ii) the actual treatment decision or the circumstances of the actual treatment decision do not correspond to those specified in the advance decision, or

(iii) there are reasonable grounds to believe that the situation differs from those that the adult had anticipated at the time of making the advance decision and that that difference would have affected the advance decision.[76]

4.11.8 An advance decision is invalid in its entirety where:

(i) it has been withdrawn

(ii) the power to consent (or not to consent) to the treatment has subsequently been donated to a nominated proxy via a lasting power of attorney, or

(iii) the adult has done anything else clearly inconsistent with the advance decision remaining their fixed decision.[77]

4.11.9 If the advance decision is valid then it has the same effect as if the person making the advance decision had made it competently and contemporaneously in relation to the actual treatment decision.[78] Therefore, the advance decision is a legal device that moves the patient's choice through time, making it operate when it is needed and desired by the patient (*see* Section 4.9.2).

4.11.10 In practical reality, decisions must often be made with less than complete information. If the responsible medical professional reasonably believes that the advance decision is valid and that it applies to the treatment in prospect, then *there is a statutory defence to any liability that might arise from the withholding or withdrawing of the*

---

75   s 25(3) *Mental Capacity Act 2005.*
76   s 25(4) *Mental Capacity Act 2005.*
77   s 25(2) *Mental Capacity Act 2005.*
78   s 26(1) *Mental Capacity Act 2005.*

treatment.[79] Here, the word 'reasonably' imports an objective element (*see* Section 10.2).

4.11.11 Sometimes there can be uncertainty surrounding the validity of the advance decision or whether it applies to the treatment in prospect. Where this is the case *there is another statutory defence that protects from liability that might arise from continuing with the treatment.* In order for this to operate the responsible medical professional must **not** be satisfied either that the advance decision exists, or is valid, or applies to the treatment in prospect. If the responsible medical professional is satisfied that the advance decision is valid and operates then the statutory defence is not available.[80]

4.11.12 In some cases the uncertainty can be acute. For example, when it is unclear if an advance decision in relation to life-sustaining treatment has been withdrawn or not. In such cases an application can be made to the Court of Protection to resolve these issues.[81] When such uncertainty exists and the opinion of the Court is being sought, the statute permits life-sustaining treatment and any other actions necessary to prevent a serious deterioration in the patient's condition.[82]

4.12 LASTING POWERS OF ATTORNEY: GENERAL

4.12.1 According to the *Concise Oxford English Dictionary* the word 'attorney' is derived from Old French, meaning to turn towards. In modern times it has come to mean someone who has been appointed by another to act on their behalf. Originally these were people who could manage financial and property matters. Such powers for agents to manage the affairs of another potentially left the donor at risk if they became unable to supervise the agent. Therefore, these powers lapsed once the donor became incompetent.[83]

4.12.2 As time progressed it became clear that it would be desirable for these powers to have the possibility of continuing once the donor became incompetent. This is called an **Enduring Power of Attorney** and, to protect the donor, it has to be registered with the Court.[84] However,

---

79   s 26(3) *Mental Capacity Act 2005.*
80   s 26(2) *Mental Capacity Act 2005.*
81   s 26(4) *Mental Capacity Act 2005.*
82   s 26(5) *Mental Capacity Act 2005.*
83   *Drew v Nunn* (1879) 4 QB 661.
84   *Enduring Powers of Attorney Act 1985.*

Enduring Powers of Attorney cover only financial and property affairs.

4.12.3   The *Mental Capacity Act 2005* introduces **Lasting Powers of Attorney (LPA)**. These persist after the donor becomes incompetent and can operate both in relation to property matters and in relation to matters of personal welfare, including giving or withholding consent to medical treatments.[85,86]

4.12.4   Enduring Powers of Attorney that already exist are preserved and the legal machinery governing them is absorbed within the *Mental Capacity Act 2005*.[87] However, no further Enduring Powers of Attorney can be created.[88] All newly created powers of attorney will be Lasting Powers of Attorney.

4.12.5   Lasting Powers of Attorney must comply with a prescribed form[89] and will have to be registered with the Office of the Public Guardian (*see* Section 4.8.9).

4.13   LASTING POWERS OF ATTORNEY: DECISIONS OVER PERSONAL WELFARE

4.13.1   The situation is complex. Therefore, we will only consider here the powers that the donee of a Lasting Power of Attorney may exercise in relation to important medical decisions, as these are likely to be the most commonly arising issues in modern medical practice. There are additional specific provisions for managing financial and property affairs, and for balancing the liberty of the incompetent donee where some form of physical restraint is required.[90]

4.13.2   The power granted by a donor of a Lasting Power of Attorney to the donee can include the power to give or refuse consent to medical treatment.[91] The powers donated can be restricted by the instrument creating the power.[92] The transferred power does not cover life-preserving treatments unless this additional power is

---

85   s 9(1) and 11(7)(c) *Mental Capacity Act 2005*.
86   para. 7.21 Code of Practice *Mental Capacity Act 2005*. www.publicguardian.gov.uk.
87   s 66(3) and Schedule 4 *Mental Capacity Act 2005*.
88   s 66(2) *Mental Capacity Act 2005*.
89   Schedule 1 *Mental Capacity Act 2005*. A draft form is presently available from the Department of Constitutional Affairs website: www.dca.gov.uk.
90   *See* Code of Practice *Mental Capacity Act 2005*. www.guardianship.gov.uk.
91   s 11(7)(c) *Mental Capacity Act 2005*.
92   s 9(4)(b) *Mental Capacity Act 2005*.

explicitly transferred by the instrument creating the lasting power of attorney.[93]

4.13.3 The powers of the donee of a Lasting Power of Attorney are subject to the same limitations as apply to a decision made by an advance directive. Thus a decision can be expressed in lay terms, and the same protections apply to questions surrounding the validity of the Lasting Power of Attorney or whether it applies to the medical decision under consideration. Similarly, an application can be made to the Court of Protection for a ruling (*see* Sections 4.11.10–4.11.12).

4.13.4 It is not entirely clear from the Guidance whether the exercise of a valid Lasting Power of Attorney in refusing life-sustaining treatment must be in writing.[94] Given the gravity of the decision, the best approach is likely to be to obtain such a refusal in writing.

4.13.5 The theory is that the decision-making power (*see* paras. 3.1.3–3.1.4) of the donor should be maximised. Therefore, when the donor has capacity to make their own decision neither an advance decision nor an authorised proxy decision-maker has power to make the decision.[95]

4.13.6 Where a valid advance decision is executed after the donation of a Lasting Power of Attorney, the advance decision operates. However, if the advance decision precedes the creation of the Lasting Power of Attorney then the advance decision is deemed revoked by the Lasting Power of Attorney.[96] Confusion might arise where both are executed on the same day, in which case they should be dated and the time of execution noted.

4.13.7 A key advantage of decision making by a proxy chosen in advance by the patient is the fact that the patient's values and preferences are more likely to be expressed in decisions made by this chosen proxy. The disadvantage is that the decision-making is two steps removed from the donor making the decision contemporaneously himself.

4.13.8 The first step is the separation in time of the donor's decision and its implementation. The proxy's power does not operate while the patient has capacity.

---

93   s 11(8) *Mental Capacity Act 2005.*
94   ss 11(7)(b) and 25(6) *Mental Capacity Act 2005.*
95   ss 11(7)(a) and 24(1) and *Mental Capacity Act 2005.*
96   ss 25(2), (7) *Mental Capacity Act 2005 .*

4.13.9   The second is that, unlike an advance decision, the donor can only
          select the proxy, not make the decision themselves. This creates a
          problem. How can the power of the proxy be restrained from misuse?
          The solution is to constrain the power available to the proxy by the
          best interests test.[97] Additionally, the exercise of the power of the
          proxy cannot be motivated by a desire to bring about the death of the
          donor.[98]

4.13.10   The proxy does not have power of consent in relation to treatments
          for a mental disorder; that is given under the provisions of the *Mental
          Health Act 1983* as amended.[99] In practice, this will have greatest
          impact upon those treatments given by virtue of s 58(3)(b) *Mental
          Health Act 1983* as amended, i.e. on the basis of a second medical
          opinion rather than the consent of the patient.

4.13.11   It is instructive to consider how these principles might operate in
          relation to the power to refuse life-sustaining treatment.[100] Consider
          the facts of *St George's Healthcare NHS Trust v S*[101] (*see* Section 4.5.3).
          Here P was suffering life-threatening pre-eclampsia but refusing a life-
          saving caesarean section. If P was incompetent but had made a valid
          advance decision covering the circumstances (she had in fact refused
          her consent clearly and in writing), then the advance decision would
          be effective in refusing the caesarean section (*see* Section 4.11.9).

4.13.12   If she subsequently competently executed a Lasting Power of Attorney
          donating a proxy power over the decision, then her advance directive
          would lapse (*see* Section 4.11.8). In this situation, the proxy could
          give their consent to the life-saving caesarean section because it
          was in her best interests. Conversely, if a valid advance decision was
          executed after the donation of the Lasting Power of Attorney, then
          the donee and the responsible medical professional would be bound
          by the advance decision.[96] In reality, it is likely that the Court would
          be called upon to determine whether the advance decision was valid
          and, if it was not valid, where P's best interests lay.[102]

4.13.13   Where two or more persons act as donees of a Lasting Power of
          Attorney, they must act jointly unless the legal instrument creating
          the Lasting Power of Attorney allows them to act independently

---

97   s 9(4) *Mental Capacity Act 2005*.
98   s 4(5) *Mental Capacity Act 2005*.
99   s 28 *Mental Capacity Act 2005*.
100   s 11(8) *Mental Capacity Act 2005*.
101   [1998] 3 All ER 673.
102   ss 22, 23 *Mental Capacity Act 2005*.

(severally). This means that in the absence of a term in the legal document granting the donees the power to act independently the decisions of the donees are not effective unless they are all agreed.[103]

4.13.14 As a final observation under this heading, note that a bankrupt cannot be appointed as the donee of a Lasting Power of Attorney in relation to financial and property matters.[104] No such restrictions apply to matters of medical welfare.

4.14 INDEPENDENT MENTAL CAPACITY ADVOCATES (IMCAS)

4.14.1 Independent mental capacity advocates work to represent and support incompetent adults (*see* Section 4.8.2), including those with mental disorders.[105] IMCAs must be involved,[106] inter alia, where the patient is about to receive 'serious medical treatment'[107] and there is no one appropriate, other than paid carers or professionals, to consult in relation to determining where the patient's best interests lie.

4.14.2 Serious medical treatment refers to situations where:

(i) there is a fine balance between the risks and benefits of a proposed treatment

(ii) there is a choice of treatments, and

(iii) the decision as to which treatment option is best is finely balanced *or* the proposed treatment may involve serious consequences for the patient.[108]

4.14.3 If the medical situation demands urgent treatment then this can be delivered even if the IMCA has not been instructed.[109]

4.14.4 IMCAs can also be involved in the review of accommodation arrangements and in adult protection cases,[110] and they can have a role in

---

103 s 10(5) *Mental Capacity Act 2005*.
104 s 10(2) *Mental Capacity Act 2005*.
105 ss 130A–130D *Mental Health Act 1983* as amended.
106 s 37(3) *Mental Capacity Act 2005*. Save in emergencies or in relation to treatment under Part 4 of the *Mental Health Act 1983*.
107 s 37 *Mental Capacity Act 2005*, para. 4 The *Mental Capacity Act 2005 (Independent Mental Capacity Advocates) (General) Regulations 2006* SI 2006/1832.
108 s 37 *Mental Capacity Act 2005*.
109 s 37(4) *Mental Capacity Act 2005*.
110 *Mental Capacity Act 2005 (Independent Mental Capacity Advocates) (Expansion of Role) Regulations 2006* SI 2006/2883.

supporting decision-making in cases where a patient's liberty may be deprived.[111]

4.14.5   Once involved in the care of the patient, the responsibilities of the IMCA involve collecting information relevant to the decision in prospect and preparing a report for the person instructing them. The collection of information may involve interviewing the patient, examining the medical records, and consulting those caring for the patient and other relevant persons.[112]

4.14.6   The IMCA has the power to challenge any decision made as an interested party.[113] The impact of such challenges will be determined to a great extent by how frequent and appropriate such challenges are in practice.

4.14.7   There is a great danger that IMCAs will simply rubber stamp medical decision-making. Time will tell if the service in fact develops as a powerful and effective safeguard for the best interests of this group of vulnerable adults.

---

111 s 39A *Mental Capacity Act 2005.*

112 *Mental Capacity Act 2005 (Independent Mental Capacity Advocates) (General) Regulations 2006* SI 2006/1832 para. 4.

113 *Mental Capacity Act 2005 (Independent Mental Capacity Advocates) (General) Regulations 2006* SI 2006/1832 para. 7.

5 Consent: children

5.1 THE TEST FOR CAPACITY: CHILDREN

5.1.1 Children are not born with capacity but, as they grow, most will achieve capacity over time. The age of majority is 18 years.[1] Between the ages of 16 and 18 years there is a presumption that a child has capacity to give consent to procedures involving medical diagnosis or treatment.[2]

5.1.2 For other decisions in children aged 16–18 years,[3] and all decisions for children below the age of 16 years, the question of when a child has capacity in relation to a particular decision was addressed in the leading case of *Gillick v West Norfolk and Wisbech Area Health Authority* (*see* Section 5.3.1).[4] This case decided that a child below the age of 16 years can offer valid consent to a medical treatment when the child achieves a *sufficient understanding and intelligence* to enable them to make an informed decision in relation to the proposed medical treatment.[5] Such a child is said to be *Gillick* competent.

5.1.3 For a child, unlike adults, implicit in the test of capacity is the need to demonstrate understanding of the risks and benefits of the proposed treatment. This additional requirement makes it harder for children to establish capacity.

5.1.4 The standard of intelligence and depth of understanding required from the child is relative to the gravity of the particular choice to be made. For example, in *Re: S (a minor)(consent to medical treatment)*

---

1   s 1 *Family Law Reform Act 1969*.
2   s 8 *Family Law Reform Act 1969* – note this has been interpreted as not granting the right to refuse treatment: *Re: W* [1992] 4 All ER 627.
3   Note that valid *Gillick* competence still operates for children aged 16–18 years: s 8(3) *Family Law Reform Act 1969*.
4   *Gillick v West Norfolk and Wisbech Area Health Authority* [1985] 3 All ER 402.
5   Note that section 2(a) *Mental Capacity Act 2005* states that capacity cannot be established merely by reference to a person's age. It is possible that this provision may impact upon the common law test for competence in children but not the other rules surrounding consent in children. This is because the powers that can be exercised under the *Mental Capacity Act* can be exercised in relation to persons under the age of 16 years: s 5(b) *Mental Capacity Act 2005*.

(*see* Section 5.4.4), in order for P to be *Gillick* competent she would have had to demonstrate 'a greater understanding of the manner of the death' and the associated 'pain and distress'.

5.1.5   For an adult, once the test of capacity (*see* Section 4.1.1) has been satisfied and the patient has been adequately informed of the risks and benefits of the proposed treatment, then a freely expressed refusal of consent is valid. The adult must demonstrate that they *can* understand the decision but they do not need to *demonstrate* that they do understand the decision. The presumption in favour of capacity possessed by adults appears to have impact here. It can be displaced, for example, where there is a disturbance of impairment in the functioning of their mind, then the burden to establish capacity in adults is greater.[6]

5.1.6   Children lack this presumption of capacity. Therefore, where irrevocable harm may result from the decision, it seems that more is demanded from the child than an adult in a similar situation before a valid refusal of consent to the proposed treatment is respected. It may be that the greater the magnitude of the risk, the greater the depth of understanding of the situation the child needs to display before they can possess *Gillick* competence.

5.1.7   In order to give valid consent, the child should have sufficient understanding and intelligence in relation to the proposed treatment to understand its nature and purpose, the associated risks and benefits, and the available alternatives.

5.2   PARENTAL RESPONSIBILITY AND THE JURISDICTION OF THE COURT: CHILDREN

5.2.1   Children are subject to certain protections within society. People vested with parental responsibility have duties to protect their children and the Court has special jurisdiction in relation to children.[7]

5.2.2   People with parental responsibility have the power to consent to treatment on behalf of the child.[8,9,10,11] A birth mother gains parental

---

6   *Re: C* [1994] 1 All ER 819.
7   *Gillick v West Norfolk and Wisbech Area Health Authority* [1985] 3 All ER 402.
8   s 3(1) *Children Act 1989.*
9   *Re: Z (a minor) (freedom of publication)* [1995] 4 All ER 961, 979 per Ward LJ.
10   *Re: R (a minor) (wardship: medical treatment)* [1991] 4 All ER 177 per Lord Donaldson MR.
11   Re: *K, W and H (minors) (medical treatment)* [1993] 1 FLR 854 – compulsory psychiatric treatment ruled legal on the basis of parental consent alone.

responsibility upon the birth of the child.[12] A father gains parental responsibility if he:

(i) is married to the mother at the time of the child's birth[13]

(ii) jointly registers the child's birth with the mother

(iii) makes a parental responsibility agreement with the mother, or

(iv) is granted parental responsibility by court order.[14]

5.2.3 Other people or bodies may also possess parental responsibility including appointed guardians,[15] people who obtain a residence order[16] and the Local Authority.[17] A person who has care of the child but lacks parental responsibility may do what is necessary to safeguard the welfare of the child.[18]

5.2.4 Where more than one person has parental responsibility over the child each can act independently but must act to safeguard the welfare of the child.[19] There are certain situations, e.g. circumcision[20] and immunisation,[21] which require the consent of both parents.

5.2.5 The Court has an inherent jurisdiction over the welfare of children. The powers exercisable under this *parens patriae* jurisdiction[22] are theoretically limitless.[23] The Court also has the power to permit or refuse to permit treatment where the child is a ward of court,[24] or by issuing a 'specific issue order' or a 'prohibited steps order'.[25]

---

12 s 2 *Children Act 1989*; s 27(1) *Human Fertilisation and Embryology Act 1990*.
13 s 2(1) *Children Act 1989*.
14 s 4(1) *Children Act 1989*.
15 s 5(6) *Children Act 1989*.
16 s 12(2)*Children Act 1989*.
17 Care order: s 33(3)(b) *Children Act 1989*; Emergency protection order: s 44(4)(c) *Children Act 1989*.
18 s 3(5) *Children Act 1989*.
19 s 2(7) *Children Act 1989*.
20 *Re: J (specific issue orders: child's religious upbringing and circumcision)* [2000] 1 FLR 571.
21 *Re: C (welfare of child: immunisation)* [2003] EWCA Civ 1148.
22 The *parens patriae* jurisdiction – see *Re: Z (a minor) (freedom of publication)* [1995] 4 All ER 961, 966 per Ward LJ.
23 For example, they can be used to order a child to be detained for medical treatment: *Re: C (detention: medical treatment)* [1997] 2 FLR 180.
24 The major practical distinction between wardship and the inherent jurisdiction is that, for a ward of court, no important step in the life of that child can be taken without the consent of the court. Wardship is not available for children under the care of a local authority: section 100(2)(c) *Children Act 1989*.
25 s 8 *Children Act 1989*.

5.3   *GILLICK* COMPETENCE

5.3.1   Where a child is *Gillick* competent and does offer their informed and voluntary consent to the proposed medical treatment then such consent is sufficient legal justification to permit the treatment to be lawfully delivered. People with parental responsibility cannot remove this legal justification.[4] This last point is important and exemplified by the facts of the famous *Gillick* case.

Gillick v West Norfolk and Wisbech Area Health Authority [1985] 3 All ER 402, HL

Fraser Ld, Scarmen Ld, Bridge Ld, Brandon Ld, Templeman Ld

P was the mother of five girls aged under 16 years. The Department of Health and Social Security issued a circular advising that if a doctor was consulted in a family planning clinic by a girl aged less than 16 years it would not be unlawful for the doctor to prescribe contraceptives for the girl without the knowledge or consent of her parents.

P sought, inter alia, a declaration that the advice was unlawful.

Held: It was not unlawful for a doctor acting in accordance with their *bona fide* clinical judgement to prescribe contraceptives for a girl under the age of 16 years.

Parental rights derived from the parental duty to protect their child. These rights recede as the child develops sufficient intelligence and understanding to reach their own conclusions on the issue.

5.3.2   An alternative approach by a parent seeking to exercise control over this decision in relation to their *Gillick* competent child was made by attacking the duty of confidentiality (*see* Section 2) owed by the medical professional to the child. The attack was unsuccessful, meaning that the parent cannot invade the duty of confidence owed by a medical professional to a *Gillick* competent child using the power of their parental responsibility alone.[26]

---

26   *R v Secretary of State for Health ex parte Axon* [2006] EWHC 37. *See,* also, Bridgeman J. Young people and sexual health: whose rights? Whose responsibilities? *R. (on the application of Axon) v Secretary of State for Health & another. Med Law Rev.* 2006; **14**(3): 418–24.

5.3.3   Similarly, where the child is a ward of the Court the welfare of the child remains the paramount concern of the Court and forms the basis of the respect for the child's decision.

Re: P [1986] 1 FLR 272, Fam

P was a 15-year-old girl who was a ward of the Court and was 11 weeks pregnant. P sought an abortion which would have been lawful under section 1(a) of the *Abortion Act 1967*. P's parents opposed this on religious grounds.

   P had gone into care after a conviction for theft when she was 13. She had already had a child when she was 14. P remained in care, was succeeding at school and was a good parent. Given she was living in a hostel, P felt she could not manage with a second child.

Held: Abortion was permitted as it best promoted P's welfare.

5.4   *GILLICK* COMPETENT CHILDREN: REFUSAL OF CONSENT

5.4.1   When a *Gillick* competent child refuses consent to a treatment, that refusal does not completely determine whether or not the treatment can be delivered.[2] The essence of the tort of battery is that it arises when there is no legal justification for a physical touching. Therefore, if another source of legal justification other than the consent of the *Gillick* competent child can be found, then it may be possible to deliver the treatment lawfully.

5.4.2   For example, where a person possessing parental responsibility gives consent,[27] then it may be possible to deliver treatment lawfully. However, parental rights are linked to and derive from parental duties. This was the view of Lord Scarmen in *Gillick*. He felt that, because parental rights arise from the parental duties, they must be exercised to promote the welfare of the child.[28] He also approved the view of Ld Denning MR in *Hewyer v Bryant*[29] where he described the parental right as 'a dwindling right' that begins 'with a right to control' and ends with little more than a right to give advice. Thus, parental rights

---

27   *Re: R* [1991] 4 All ER 177.
28   *Re: S (a minor) (consent to medical treatment)* [1994] 2 FLR 1065.
29   [1969] 3 All ER 578, 582.

were rights that the court would 'hesitate to enforce against the wishes of the child' as the child got older.

5.4.3   Therefore, when a *Gillick* competent child refuses consent to a particular treatment, the predominant question becomes where does the welfare of the child lie?[30] Ultimately this issue falls to the Court to decide. Once it has resolved this issue, the Court has the power to authorise treatment, even in situations where a *Gillick* competent child has refused consent, effectively overriding that *Gillick* competent refusal of consent.

Re: W (a minor)(medical treatment) [1992] 4 All ER 627, CA

P was a 16-year-old girl suffering from anorexia nervosa. She required naso-gastric feeding. P initially consented to naso-gastric feeding.

The local authority initially applied[31] to the Court for leave to move the minor to a named treatment unit and to treat P using naso-gastric feeding.

At first instance Thorpe J held that: (1) P was *Gillick* competent to accept naso-gastric feeding; (2) that the Court had the necessary powers to authorise the transfer and therefore authorised the transfer.

After transfer P persisted in refusing food and deteriorated medically.

An application was made to the Court of Appeal for an emergency order to enable her to be treated in specialist hospital without her consent.

Held: NG feeding ordered in best interests of the child.

It was doubted whether the child was *Gillick* competent, but the power of the Court was sufficient to override the wishes of a child who was *Gillick* competent when this was in the best interests of the child. The Court could authorise the doctors to undertake the necessary treatment in accordance with their clinical judgement.

Section 8 of the Family Law Reform Act 1969 (*see* para. 5.1.1) permitted consent to treatment but did not operate to permit P to refuse the treatment. Such treatment could be delivered where another legal justification could be found.

5.4.4   The power of the Court is sufficient to override the refusal of consent to treatment by those holding parental responsibility where this will

---

30   s 1 *Children Act 1989.*
31   Under s 100(3) *Children Act 1989,* for exercise by the Court of the inherent jurisdiction.

promote the welfare of the child. In *Re: S (a minor) (consent to medical treatment)*[32] the child was found to be *Gillick* incompetent but it is likely that the outcome would have been the same if P had been found to be *Gillick* competent.

Re: S (a minor)(consent to medical treatment)[1994] 2 FLR 1065

P was a 15½-year-old girl suffering from beta minor thalassemia. She was also a Jehovah's Witness. She required and had been receiving frequent transfusion and desferroxamine infusions.

P rejected further treatment. She retained a belief that a miracle may save her. P's parents were also Jehovah's Witnesses, and supported P's decision. The Local Authority invoked the court's inherent jurisdiction.

Held: P was not *Gillick* competent to refuse live-saving treatment. Her capacity was not commensurate with the gravity of the decision. Declaration granted that continued treatment was lawful as it was in P's best interests.[33]

5.4.5   Notice that if the Court determines that a particular treatment option lies in the best interests of a child it does not matter whether the child is *Gillick* competent or not. The Court can authorise the treatment in either case. However, the views of the child are likely to be given greater weight if they are *Gillick* competent.

5.4.6   On the acute and serious facts of *Re: M*[34] the Court did not formally consider whether the child was *Gillick* competent or not.

Re: M [1999] 2 FLR 1097

M was a competent 15½-year-old girl who sustained severe heart failure and required a heart transplant. She stated that she did not want someone else's heart and refused to give consent.

Held: It was in her best interests to have the transplant.

---

32   *Re: S (a minor) (consent to medical treatment)* [1994] 2 FLR 1065.
33   If competent, then because death would ensue, the Court would have to operate best interests to preserve life of child. (per Andrew Grubb in commentary [1996] 4 *Med L Rev* 84).
34   [1999] 2 FLR 1097.

5.4.7   Religious values should not impact on the question of *Gillick* competence.[35] However in some cases it seems that the question of whether a
child is *Gillick* competent or not can become infused with the separate
question about whether the child's best interests lie with receiving the
treatment or not. In situations where there are sincerely held beliefs
sometimes only a tragic choice exists. With the benefit of hindsight, we
must recognise that there are times when respect for the autonomous
decision of a *Gillick* competent child must remain a serious option.[36]

Re: E (a minor) [1993] 1 FLR 386

P was a 15¾-year-old Jehovah's Witness who suffered acute leukaemia.
In order to receive treatment with a 80–90% chance of complete remission,
he required a blood transfusion. Without the blood transfusion his chances
of complete remission were only 40–50%.

P refused blood transfusion. P's parents supported P's decision.

Held: P was not *Gillick* competent. The transfusion was authorised.

When P reached 18 years he competently refused consent to further
transfusions and died.[37]

5.4.8   Was the child in *Re: E (a minor)*[38] really *Gillick* incompetent? Some
children are sufficiently mature to understand fully the decision and
are capable of making a choice that, for them, is the right one. The
tragedy in *Re: E (a minor)* (para. 5.4.7) was that the child meant what
he said and could only demonstrate this once he had reached full
adulthood.

5.4.9   For this reason, if not for any other, it seems correct that the Court
should clearly separate the question of whether a child is *Gillick*
competent from the question of where the child's welfare lies. This
approach might help to keep alive the possibility that respect for
a *Gillick* competent child's refusal of life-preserving treatment is a
genuine possibility even where this might lead to a medically adverse
outcome. One option may be to develop rules that distinguish a sub-
group of 'mature minors' whose decisions may carry sufficient force
to refuse life-saving treatments.[36]

---

35   *Re: W (a minor) (medical treatment)* [1992] 4 All ER 627, 637d per Lord Donaldson MR.
36   *See In Re: EG* (1989) 549 NE 2d 322, Illinois Sup Ct.
37   McHale J, Tingle J. *Law and Nursing.* 2nd ed. Butterworths-Heinemann; 2001. p. 119.
38   [1993] 1 FLR 386.

5.4.10   Notice the difference between the ongoing treatment required in *Re: E (a minor)*[39] the one-off treatment needed in *Re: L (medical treatment: Gillick competency)*[40] (para. 5.5.3). The need for ongoing treatment may be an additional important factor in any determination of where the welfare of the child lies.

5.5   *GILLICK* INCOMPETENT CHILDREN

5.5.1   The general powers of the *Mental Capacity Act 2005* do apply to children aged of 16 years or above.[41] However the power to create advance directives[42] and lasting powers of attorney[43] does not become available until the age of 18 years.

5.5.2   For *Gillick* incompetent children consent must come from those holding parental responsibility or the Court (*see* Section 5.2). Other justifications such as emergency can also operate. We have seen that parental rights are constrained by the welfare of the child (*see* Section 5.4.2).

5.5.3   Differing opinions can exist between the parents and the medical professionals,[44] between the parents themselves[45] and, on occasion, the parents and medical professionals may agree but differ from the opinion of the Court.[46] When there is an intractable conflict between the views of the parent and the views of the medical professionals in relation to the care of an incompetent child the view of the Court should be sought,[47] urgently if necessary (*see* Section 5.5.2).

5.5.4   The Court is bound to promote the welfare of the child.[48] In order to do this it can look to where the best interests of the child lie.[49] The Court exercises its own judgement. It does not seek to determine whether the parents, the medical professionals or other involved parties views are strongest.[50]

---

39   [1992] 2 FCR 219.
40   [1998] 2 FLR 810.
41   s 2(5)(b) *Mental Capacity Act 2005*.
42   s 24(1) *Mental Capacity Act 2005*.
43   s 9(2)(c) *Mental Capacity Act 2005*.
44   *R v Portsmouth Hospital NHS Trust* ex parte *Glass* [1999] EWCA Civ 1914.
45   *Re: C (welfare of Child: immunisation)* [2003] EWCA Civ 1148.
46   For example, *Re: B (a minor) (wardship: medical treatment)* (1981) [1990] 3 All ER 927.
47   *R v Portsmouth Hospital NHS Trust* ex parte *Glass* [1999] EWCA Civ 1914.
48   s 1 *Children Act 1989*.
49   *Re: MB* (1997) 8 Med LR 217, 225 per Butler-Sloss LJ.
50   *Re: A (children) (conjoined twins: surgical separation)* [2000] 4 All ER 961, 1055 per Robert Walker LJ.

5.5.5   The failure of medical professionals to respect an effective refusal of consent can constitute a breach of the Article 8 right to a private life under the *Human Rights Act 1998*. This has been interpreted to operate to protect a right to physical integrity which supports the negative aspects (the shield) of the right to self-determination.

R v Portsmouth Hospital NHS Trust ex parte *Glass* [1999] EWCA Civ 1914

P was a 12-year-old old boy suffering from severe mental and physical disabilities. These included cerebral palsy, hydrocephalus, epilepsy, impaired cognitive function and visual handicap.

On 9 July 1998 P was admitted to the intensive care unit after a tonsillectomy. There he suffered recurrent infections. Opiates were initially used to control pain. He was discharged home on 2 September 1998.

After several readmissions, P was once again readmitted on 18 October 1998. The doctors believed that P was dying but the mother refused to accept this view. On 20 October 1998 an opiate infusion was started despite the mother's explicit refusal of consent to the use of opiates.

The depth of the disagreement was evidenced by a violent incident on the 21 October 1998, resulting in two members of the medical staff sustaining injuries.[51] P was subsequently discharged and improved with antibiotics and a change of feeding regime.

P sought judicial review of the clinical decision.

Scott-Baker J, at first instance, held that judicial review is a blunt tool for this type of action, exercise of discretion *ex post facto* would not alter the situation, and relief was denied.

Held CA: No grounds to interfere with the discretion of Scott-Baker J. If future irreconcilable conflicts occur, then the parties should apply to the Court for resolution through the short-notice, best interests procedure.

P appealed to the European Court of Human Rights (ECHR).

ECHR held in 2004:[52] There was unjustified breach of P's Article 8: right to respect for his private life.

This right encompasses P's right to physical integrity. 10 000 euros damages was awarded, plus costs.

---

51   Three people were convicted of causing actual bodily harm and violent disorder in consequence.
52   *Glass v United Kingdom* [2004] ECHR 103.

The ECHR had previously rejected the suggestion that doctors had intended to hasten P's death through the use of the diamorphine. Thus P's article 2: right to life was not breached.

P's mother was acting as P's legal proxy. The failure to respect P's mother's refusal of consent to treatment with diamorphine invaded P's right to physical integrity. On the particular facts of the case this invasion was not necessary given that an application to the Court could have been used to assess where P's best interests lay.

5.5.6   It is unclear if the right to physical integrity is coterminous with the right to be free from unjustified physical interference. Even if not precisely coterminous, they are likely to accord closely in practice.

5.5.7   When parents seek to withhold their consent in a way that reflects their personal values, this may conflict with where the Court subsequently determines the child's best interests lie. In this situation the Court can override the parents' views.

Re: D (a minor) (wardship: medical treatment) (1981) [1990] 3 All ER 927, CA

P was a 10-day-old girl suffering Down's syndrome. P suffered an 'intestinal blockage'[53] that would be fatal if not surgically treated. P's parents refused consent to the surgery. Their view was that 'God or nature had given the child a way out'.

Held: P should have the operation.

The test applied was whether, as a result of the Down's syndrome, the child's life was destined to be so demonstrably awful that the child should be condemned to die. The answer here was no.

5.5.8   The same principle operates where the parental objection to treatment is based on religious grounds rather than personal values[54] (*see* also Sections 19.12.9–19.12.11).

---

53   Presumably duodenal atresia.
54   An American judge, Rutledge J (*Prince v Massachusetts* (1944) 321 US 158,170) using language more appropriate to 1944, declared that 'parents are free to become martyrs themselves, but it does not follow that they are free in identical circumstances to make martyrs of their children . . .'.

Re: S (a minor)(medical treatment)[1993] 1 FLR 376, Fam, Thorpe J

P was a 4½-year-old child suffering from T-cell leukaemia and requiring intensive chemotherapy. Transfusion of blood or blood products was essential for the treatment of chemotherapy to have any chance of success.

P's parents were Jehovah's Witnesses and opposed the transfusions.

Held: Transfusion permitted.

The argument that the family as the unit would suffer if the child received a blood transfusion in the face of the parental wishes was considered. On the evidence it appeared the family would accept that the responsibility for consent had been taken from them.

5.5.9 Similarly, in *Re: O (a minor) (medical treatment)*[55] P was a 10-day-old baby born 12 weeks prematurely and weighing only 1.28 kg. She was suffering from respiratory distress syndrome. Blood transfusions were required to treat the child but were refused by the parents who were Jehovah's Witnesses. The Court permitted the necessary transfusions.

5.5.10 In *NHS Trust v A (a child)*[56] the child was 6 months old and suffering haemophagocytic lymphohistiocytosis (HLH). She was a candidate for therapeutic bone marrow transplantation. The quoted procedural risks were 50% cure, 10% survival with treatment but with significant impairment, 30% unsuccessful treatment with death and 10% mortality. The child was well enough to be living at home with her parents. The parents objected to this and asked the Court to permit the child to be allowed to die without suffering the pain and distress of the treatment. The Court declared that the bone marrow treatment would be lawful in the best interests of the child, despite the objections of the parents.

5.5.11 Despite these results the Court will not always override the views of the parents in all cases.

Re: T (a minor) (wardship: medical treatment) [1997] 1 All ER 906, CA

P was 18 months old and suffering from biliary atresia. At 3½ weeks old P

---

55   (1993) 4 Med LR 272.
56   [2007] EWHC 1696 (Fam).

had undergone unsuccessful and distressing hepatoportoenterostomy – a type of bilioenteric reconstruction (Kasai procedure). P now required liver transplantation in order to stand a chance of survival.

P's parents were healthcare workers. They refused consent to the liver transplant.

D felt that it was in P's best interests to receive the liver transplant but that, in order for the treatment to succeed, maternal cooperation was required for the post transplant care.

Connell J, at first instance, granted a declaration in favour of transplantation.

Held: It was not in best interests of the child to allow the procedure to proceed. Without the cooperation of the parents the procedure was unlikely to benefit the child.

5.5.12   Where people with parental responsibility disagree between themselves about whether a particular course of action is in the child's best interests the Court will look to the child's welfare.[57] The particular course of action in issue is material to the conclusion. Therefore, in such cases, immunisation[58] and testing for HIV status have been approved whilst male circumcision has not.[59]

5.5.13   The Court will also look to the welfare of the child where third parties challenge a particular course of action.

Re: D (a minor) (wardship: sterilisation) [1976] 1 All ER 326, QBD

P was an 11-year-old girl with Sotos syndrome which includes epilepsy, generalised clumsiness, an unusual facial appearance and behaviour problems. She had an IQ of 80 but was felt to be capable of marriage in due course. Her parents had agreed with D that P should be sterilised when she reached about 18 years of age as she was unlikely to be able to care for a child.

P reached puberty aged 10 years. She demonstrated no interest in the opposite sex and her opportunities in this direction were virtually non-existent. P's parents and D decided that P should be sterilised for non-therapeutic reasons overriding the views of other involved professionals.

---

57   *Re: C (HIV test)* [1993] 2 FLR 1004.
58   *Re: B (a child) (immunisation: parental rights)* [2003] EWCA Civ 1148.
59   *Re: J (child's religious upbringing and circumcision)* [1999] 2 FLR 678.

An educational psychologist brought the action seeking to prevent the sterilisation. D maintained that the decision lay within a doctor's clinical judgement.

Held: Non-therapeutic sterilisation not permitted.

5.5.14 Conversely in *Re: B (a minor) (wardship: sterilisation)*[60] an application for approval of sterilisation of an incompetent, mentally handicapped and epileptic 17-year-old girl was supported by the parents and medical evidence but opposed strongly by the Official Solicitor. The Court looked to the welfare of the girl and approved the sterilisation.[61]

5.5.15 When the *Gillick* incompetent child is refusing treatment their welfare remains the paramount question. Given this, their views, whilst not being determinative, may carry some weight nevertheless.

Re: L (medical treatment: Gillick competency) [1998] 2 FLR 810, Fam

Sir Stephen Brown P

P was a 14-year-old Jehovah's Witness with sincere religious convictions and who was mature for her age. P required a blood transfusion after suffering severe burns in a bathing accident. She had 54% burns of which 40% were full-thickness burns.

P refused. When 12 years old she had signed an advance medical directive refusing transfusions, and had renewed this two months earlier. Her parents supported her decision.

Held: P not *Gillick* competent in relation to the decision at hand. Transfusion authorised.

P's lack of capacity in relation to this decision may have been reduced by her 'limited experience of life'.[62]

5.5.16 Once a child reaches adulthood their own views come to carry sufficient weight to determine the outcome as we have seen in *Re: E (a minor)*[63] (*see* Section 5.4.7).

---

60   [1987] 2 All ER 206, HL.
61   Similarly in *Re: W (mental patient) (sterilisation)* [1993] 1 FLR 381.
62   Compare this to *Re: E (a minor)* [1993] 1 FLR 386.
63   *Re: E (a minor)* [1993] 1 FLR 386.

6 Consent and information

6.1 INTRODUCTION

6.1.1 In order for consent as an expression of the interest in self-determination to be valid, the person giving consent must be aware of the choices they face. They must have some grasp of the paths available and the risks/benefits associated with each available path. Importantly, the legal duty of a doctor has been held to extend to accurately imparting information but not to ensuring that it has been understood.[1] This should be distinguished from any professional obligation.

6.1.2 There are two aspects to understanding a treatment option.

(i) The first is understanding the actual *nature and purpose* of the treatment. For example, the mechanical fact that a coronary angiogram involves pushing a needle through the skin to place a plastic sheath and then using plastic catheters, radiation and radio-opaque contrast to image the coronary arteries.

(ii) The second aspect is understanding why *you* should have a coronary angiogram. You would need to understand the *risks, benefits and costs* of having the procedure versus the same calculation for not having the procedure. The risk/benefit information builds upon the nature/purpose information.

6.1.3 Information can be less than is required, misleading or incorrect. For the purposes of our discussion, let us encompass all these with the term 'misinformation'.

6.1.4 The law draws a distinction between the nature/purpose information and the risk/benefit information. A failure to disclose the necessary nature/purpose information, either intentionally or unintentionally, invalidates the consent.[2] In the absence of consent, an action for battery (*see* Section 3.2) is likely to succeed.

---

1   *Al Hamwi v (1) Johnston (2) North West London Hospitals NHS Trust* [2005] EWHC 206.
2   *Chatterton v Gerson* [1981] 1 All ER 257; Approved in *Sidaway v Bethlem Royal Hospital Governors* [1984] 1 All ER 1018, CA per Lord Donaldson MR. ([1985] 1 All ER 643, HL) and Lord Donaldson MR in *Freeman v Home Office (No. 2)* [1984] 1 All ER 1036.

6.1.5   By contrast, misinformation in relation to risk/benefit does not necessarily make the consent invalid and so a defence to an action for battery can be maintained. However, this does not preclude an action for negligence where the misinformation amounts to a breach of the duty to give sufficient information for a patient to reach a conclusion about whether they wish to accept the treatment or not[3] (*see* Section 6.4).

Chatterton v Gerson [1981] 1 All ER 257, QBD

P was aged 55 years. She underwent elective nylon darn repair of a small right inguinal hernia. This was complicated by entrapment of the ileo-inginal nerve associated with severe chronic pain. The site was surgically re-explored twice. The ileo-inguinal nerve was cut during the first re-exploration. The pain remained unrelieved. P was referred to a pain-specialist, D.

D performed several successful test intrathecal injections using the local anaesthetic marcaine together with adrenaline. The pain returned after about 48 hours on each occasion.

It was then decided to use phenol and glycerine as a neurolytic. This was injected intrathecally at the level of T9/10 on two occasions. Despite initial success P's pain subsequently returned. She also suffered from motor weakness in the right lower limb and complete loss of sensation in the right leg and foot.

P claimed she had not been informed of the risk of suffering power and/or sensory loss in her lower limbs as a result of the injections.

Held: P could not recover damages.

P was aware of the nature and purpose of the injections. On the evidence, D had given P sufficient information prior to the injections to discharge the duty to inform the patient of the risks and benefits associated with the injections.

6.2   NATURE AND PURPOSE

6.2.1   The legal action of battery sits close to the boundary between the civil law (which deals with questions of compensation between individuals) and the criminal law (which deals with punishment for offences

---

3   *Chatterton v Gerson* [1981] 1 All ER 257; Approved in *Sidaway v Bethlem Royal Hospital Governors* [1984] 1 All ER 1018, CA per Lord Donaldson MR. ([1985] 1 All ER 643, HL) and Lord Donaldson MR in *Freeman v Home Office (No. 2)* [1984] 1 All ER 1036.

against society). Apparent consent can obtained without the person giving the apparent consent being aware of the nature and purpose of the act to which they acquiesce. Such apparent consent has no legal effect. It can not, therefore, operate as a defence. Such ineffective consent can, in some cases, result in criminal charges being brought.

6.2.2   Fraud as to the nature or purpose of the act is sufficient to negate any apparent consent.[4] The following two old cases illustrate this point.

R v Flattery (1877) 2 QBD 410 (Ct of crown cased reserved)[5]

D was not medically qualified. D induced his victim to have sexual intercourse with him on the basis that this might cure her of fits.

Held: The apparent consent was invalid. D was convicted of rape.[6]

R v Williams [1923] 1 KB 340 (CCA)

D was teaching a 16-year-old girl to sing. D induced the girl to have sexual intercourse with him on the basis that this was a treatment to improve the production of her voice.

Held: The apparent consent was invalid. D was convicted of rape.[7]

6.2.3   In the Canadian case of R v Harms[8] D was medically qualified and induced the victim to have sexual intercourse on the basis that this was medical treatment. D was convicted on the basis that the act was carnal not therapeutic and the victim had consented to a therapeutic act.

6.2.4   Fraud as to the identity of the actor is also sufficient to negate consent.[9] It seems that what the patient consents to is the performance of a medical act by a medically qualified practitioner.

---

4   Note that the two rape cases are now covered by s 76(2)(a) *Sexual Offences Act 2003*.
5   Compare this with *R v Case* (1850) 4 Cox CC 220.
6   *See* now s 76(2)(a) *Sexual Offences Act 2003*.
7   Note that the two rape cases are now covered by s 76(2)(a) *Sexual Offences Act 2003*.
8   (1944) 2 DLR 61, Sup Ct Can.
9   *See*, also, *R v Dica* [2004] EWCA Crim 1103, CCA where, for the offence of actual bodily harm, consent to sexual intercourse does not necessarily include consent to taking the risk of acquiring HIV, and the similar case of *R v Cuerrier* [1998] 2 S C.R. 371.

R v Navid Tabassum [2000] 2 Cr Ct App Rep 328, CCA

D was not medically qualified. He had previously worked as a medical representative in relation to breast cancer products. D induced three victims, V, to undergo breast examinations.

V believed D was medically qualified and that the examinations were for medical purposes, i.e. a breast cancer survey.

D was convicted of indecent assault. D appealed.

Held: Conviction upheld.

V had consented to a medical examination. D was not medically qualified and therefore could not have performed a medical examination. Their consent was invalid.

6.2.5   In an older, Canadian case the same result pertained in relation to an action for battery.

R v Maurantanio (1967) 61 DLR (2d) 674 (Ontario CA)

D was not medically qualified yet offered medical services for money. P received medical treatment from D. P brought an action of battery on the basis that P had not consented to treatment by a person who was not medically qualified.

Held: Action of battery succeeded.

6.2.6   If the fraud is not as to the nature of the act or the identity of the person then, for the criminal law unlike the civil law, the fraud may not negate consent.[10,11] In the next case, the fraud as to qualification to practice was held not to go to the identity of the person performing the act. One view of the case is to say that the fraud as to the qualifications induced the patient to accept the treatment but did not go to the nature or purpose of the act nor to the identity of the actor.[12] It seemed important that the relationship was a continuing one.

---

10   *See* also *De May v Roberts* (1881) 9 NW 146, Sup Ct Mich.
11   But *see Perma v Pirozzi* (1983) 457A 2d 431, New Jersey Sup Ct.
12   *See* also *Papadimitropoulos v R* (1957) 98 CLR 249, Australia High Ct.

R v Diana Richardson [1998] 2 Cr. App. R. 200, CA

D was a dentist who had been suspended from the dental register. D continued to treat patients. The patients whom D treated were not mistaken as to D's identity although they were not told D had been suspended from the dental register.

D was charged with assault occasioning actual bodily harm on the basis that the consent of D's patients had been negated by the fact that D had fraudulently induced her patients to believe that she was a registered dentist.

Held: Not guilty.

Consent was not negated unless the victim was deceived as to the act or the identity of the person performing the act.

6.2.7   In another, Canadian case the fraud as to identity was in relation to an unqualified observer. But this observer did not touch P, therefore did not invade P's interest in being free from unwanted physical interference. Whilst the doctor did invade P's rights of self-determination and privacy through the deception, the consent was valid in relation to the physical examination actually performed.

R v Bouldoc & Bird (1967) 63 DLR (2d) 82, Can Sup Ct. Hall J, Spence J

D1 was a qualified doctor who obtained consent from P to perform a vaginal examination. D1 introduced D2, a friend, as a medical student. D2 was not a medical student. P agreed to allow D2 to observe the examination. D1 competently performed the examination.

A charge of indecent assault was brought.

Held: Not guilty.

Whilst 'unethical and reprehensible' the acts performed were those consented to and fraud as to the identity of an observer was not held sufficient to negate consent to the examination.

6.3   INTENTIONAL MISINFORMATION

6.3.1   In the next case the misinformation applied both to the nature/purpose of the treatment as well as to the risks/benefits. However, the misinformation was intentionally, not merely negligently, delivered. Any apparent consent was negated by the intentional and essentially fraudulent misinformation. The action in battery succeeded with the Court awarding additional damages in the form of aggravated damages to compensate for the harm caused.

Appleton v Garrett (1997) 8 Med LR 75

D was a dentist who widely and systematically undertook unnecessary treatment for profit. Patients were fraudulently told that the work was necessary.

D had been struck off the dental register and admitted negligence.

Held: The intentional misinformation vitiated consent, hence a battery was proved. In view of the intentional bad faith, aggravated damages were awarded.

6.3.2 Where intentional misinformation is given in relation to risks/benefits alone this may be sufficient to negate consent.[13]

6.4 NEGLIGENT MISINFORMATION

6.4.1 In relation to inadvertent misinformation that is related to risk/benefit, it seems harsh to place a doctor who is striving to promote the welfare of their patient but inadvertently misquotes a percentage risk of harm in the same category as the dentist in *Appleton v Garrett*[14] (*see* Section 6.3.1). This association of the action of battery with intentional wrongdoing may, in part, explain why the Court has not permitted negligent misinformation to negate consent. Battery is effectively reserved for the more egregious cases.

6.4.2 In *Reibl v Hughes* the Court decided that unless the misinformation as to risks/benefits was intentional then the action should lie in negligence rather than in battery. Inadvertent misinformation as to risk/benefit was a breach of the medical professional's duty of care but did not destroy the validity of the consent. Notice how the intentional nature of the touching, which is at the heart of the legal action for

---

13 *Reibl v Hughes* (1980) 114 DLR (3d) 1, Can Sup Ct.
14 (1997) 8 Med LR 75.

battery, coloured the way in which the Court dealt with a question of when a defence to battery can operate.

Reibl v Hughes (1980) 114 DLR (3d) 1, Can Sup Ct.

P was 44 years old. He had to complete a further 1½ years at work in order to become eligible for a pension. He required left internal carotid endarterectomy which, in his case, carried a 10% chance of stroke and a 4% chance of death. This risk was not disclosed to P.

As a result of the procedure P suffered right-sided hemiplegia (stroke). P sued D, claiming that if he had known about the risks involved he would not have consented to the procedure.

Held: P could recover in negligence.

Where the misinformation related to the risks/benefits of the proposed treatment the consent to the treatment was valid unless the misinforming was intentionally or fraudulently done. In this case, because the misinformation was inadvertent no action lay in battery.

There was, however, a breach of the duty to adequately inform the patient about the risk/benefits of the proposed procedure, and so an action for negligence was possible.

In Canada, the information required to be given was that which the reasonable patient (see Section 10.2) with the particular characteristics of P would require before making the choice in question.[15]

6.4.3   Inadvertent non-disclosure will negate the consent for nature/purpose but, for risk/benefit, only intentional non-disclosure will negate consent. In either case, an action for negligence may still be possible.[16]

6.4.4   Given this result, it is worth considering the differences between the legal action of battery and the legal action of negligence. In battery, an intentional non-consensual touching is sufficient to bring an action. One way that we can think of this legal action is in a similar way to the way we think about negligence: as a duty, breach of that duty, and consequent damage. The duty is not to invade another's right to be free from unjustified physical interference, the breach is the unjustified intentional touching, and the consequent damage is injury to the

---

15   The modified objective test, approved in *Arndt v Smith* [1997] 2 SCR 539.
16   Somerville MA. Structuring the issues in informed consent. *McGill Law J.* 1981; **25**: 740.

protected right.[17] The breach is inevitably causally related to the injury to the protected right. Note that no tangible harm needs to result.

6.4.5   By contrast, in negligence there is a duty of care which can be inadvertently breached. This breach must be causally related to some tangible harm. This tangible harm can be injury to the person, psychiatric damage, property damage or financial damage, but the gist of the action is some form of tangible harm.

In summary, the key differences between battery and negligence are:

(i)   Battery requires unjustified touching; negligence does not.

(ii) Battery is actionable when the right to be free from unjustified touching is invaded; tangible harm is needed to sustain an action in negligence.

(iii) Battery requires an intentional breach of the protected right; in negligence the duty of care can be inadvertently breached.

(iv) There are fewer legal steps to founding an action in battery.

6.4.6   Within the context of a medical treatment there are risks that arise from the procedure itself. Such risks of adverse outcomes and side-effects are inherent within all known medical treatments. These inherent risks are distinct from those that might arise from negligent acts of the involved medical professionals.

6.4.7   In an action for negligence based on a claim that there was misinformation surrounding these inherent risks/benefits, the usual principles for an action in negligence operate. (*see* Section 8.1)

Sidaway v Bethlem Royal Hospital Governors [1985] 1 All ER 643

P was 63 years old and suffered pain in her right arm, shoulder and left forearm. D undertook C4 laminectomy and C4/5 facetectomy. There was a 1% risk of paralysis inherent in the operation because of risk to the radicular arteries supplying the spinal cord.

The operation was competently performed but the risk of paralysis materialised. P could not sue for negligent performance of the procedure,

---

17   This is not how some lawyers think about the tort. They regard the tort as complete with the intentional touching – actionable per se.

and so brought an action in negligence for failure to disclose the risk of paralysis.

Held: P could not recover. Because D had died before the trial, P was unable to establish that the 1% risk had not been disclosed.

6.4.8   *Sidaway v Bethlem Royal Hospital Governors*[18] reduced to what Lord Diplock called 'a naked question of legal principle'. There was clearly a duty to inform patients about the risks and benefits of a treatment in order to allow the patient the opportunity to decide whether or not to accept the offered treatment.[19,20] The content of this duty was 'to provide the patient with information which will enable the patient to make a balanced judgment'.[21]

6.4.9   The core legal question was: what should the yardstick for this duty be? The conclusion was that the test by which it could be determined whether the duty had been satisfied was the *Bolam* standard (Lord Diplock). This is the same standard that applies to cases of negligence relating to diagnosis and treatment. The precise information and method by which it is conveyed becomes a matter for clinical judgement, subject to this judgement being in accordance with the accepted practice of a responsible body of medical opinion (*see* Section 10.3).

Comment: This approach based on the *Bolam* standard is open to the criticism that it leaves the amount of information to be conveyed open to the medical profession rather than the Court to decide. It relies on professional integrity and professional standards to protect the underlying patient interest in self-determination.

Lord Scarmen balked at this approach. In a powerful dissent he argued for two premises:

(i)   that the yardstick for determining whether the duty of care in such cases had been met should be based on the interest that the law is seeking to protect, i.e. the patient interest in self-determination, and that

---

18   [1985] 1 All ER 643.
19   *Bolam v Friern Hospital Management Committee* [1957] 2 All ER 118.
20   *Khalid (a child) v Barnet & Chase Farm Hospital NHS Trust* [2007] EWHC 644, para. 76 per Grenfell J.
21   *Sidaway v Bethlem Royal Hospital Governors* [1985] 1 All ER 643, 665 per Templeman Ld.

(ii) the yardstick should not rest in the hands of the medical profession but in the hands of the Court.

To meet these objectives Lord Scarmen looked to the USA authorities[22] and invoked the doctrine of informed consent. This sets the standard of disclosure by what a 'reasonable patient' in the shoes of the actual patient might expect to need to know before they could make a balanced decision about the proposed treatment.

The nature of this standard is that the Court is left to determine what this reasonable patient needs to know, albeit on the basis of the medical evidence. The effect of this is to wrest the yardstick from the hands of prevailing medical practice and place it back into the hands of the Court.

The majority of the House of Lords rejected Lord Scarmen's reasoning.

6.4.10 There is, in addition, an important duty to disclose any information that the patient requests or wants to know.[23,24]

6.4.11 Beyond what was disclosed in accordance with the *Bolam* standard (i.e. a body of responsible medical practice), there is an obligation to disclose information 'that [is] so obviously necessary to an informed choice on the part of the patient that no reasonably prudent medical man would fail to make it'[25] or, in a similar vein, risks that were 'special in kind or magnitude or special to the patient'.[26] The example given of such a risk was the 10% risk of a stroke faced by the patient in *Reibl v Hughes*[27] (*see* Section 6.4.2.).

6.4.12 These 'significant risks' were reconsidered subsequently by the Court of Appeal.[28] The conclusion was that such risks should be disclosed where they would affect the judgement of a reasonable patient. Note how this result hands back some of the control over the yardstick in these cases back to the Court.

---

22   *Canterbury v Spence* (1972) 464 F 2d 772, Columbia CA.
23   *Pearce v United Bristol Healthcare NHS Trust* [1998] EWCA Civ 865.
24   *Sidaway v Bethlem Royal Hospital Governors* [1985] 1 All ER 643.
25   *Sidaway v Bethlem Royal Hospital Governors* [1985] 1 All ER 643, 662 per Lord Bridge Ld, Lord Keith.
26   *Sidaway v Bethlem Royal Hospital Governors* [1985] 1 All ER 643, 663 per Templeman Ld.
27   (1980) 114 DLR (3d) 1.
28   *Pearce v United Bristol Healthcare NHS Trust* [1998] EWCA Civ 865.

A 'reasonable patient' is a judicial conjuration that can be thought of as a typical (but hypothetical) member of the class of patients that are being informed.[29]

6.4.13　A risk that might need to be disclosed because of the particular characteristics of the patient (but not clearly to a reasonable patient) arose on the facts of the Australian case of *Rogers v Whitaker*.[30]

Rogers v Whitaker [1992] HCA 58, Aust. High Ct.

P was a competent adult who was blind in her right eye after a traumatic incident suffered when she was a child. D was an ophthalmic surgeon who undertook surgery in the right eye with the aim of improving P's sight in that eye. P was naturally concerned about any risk to her sight.

D performed the operation competently but without improvement in the vision in the right eye. As a complication of the procedure P suffered sympathetic ophthalmia in the left eye resulting in complete loss of vision in that eye.

The risk of sympathetic ophthalmia with consequent blindness was 1 in 14,000 and had not been disclosed to P prior to the operation. If P had been told of the risk she would not have undergone the surgery.

Medical evidence was that there was a reputable and responsible body of medical opinion that would not have disclosed the risk in this case.

Held: P could recover.

The Australian High Court followed a previous authority[31] and relegated the *Bolam* standard to 'a useful guide' rather than a determining standard in cases of inadvertent misinformation.

P should have been told on the basis that she had asked about any threat to her vision, albeit in layperson's terms.

6.4.14　The duty to disclose rests on the obligation that lies at the heart of the doctor–patient relationship: that is the obligation of the doctor to act to promote the welfare of the patient. Therefore, in the rare situations where the disclosure of information does not promote the welfare of

---

29　*Pearce v United Bristol Healthcare NHS Trust* [1998] EWCA Civ 865.
30　[1992] HCA 58.
31　*F v R* (1983) 33 SASR 189.

the patient, the medical professional can withhold the information as a *therapeutic privilege*.[32] This exception is narrow.

Duty to disclose – summary:

1. There is a duty to inform about the nature and purpose of the treatment, and to voluntarily disclose the inherent risks that might affect the judgement of a reasonable patient. The yardstick by which this duty is tested is the *Bolam* standard as modified by *Bolitho* (see Section 10.4).

2. There is also a duty to disclose:

   (i) risks that a patient specifically asks about

   (ii) risks which are obviously necessary to disclose, or

   (iii) are 'special in kind, magnitude or special to the patient'.

6.5   CAUSATION AND NEGLIGENT MISINFORMATION

6.5.1   Consider a patient claim for negligent misinformation: the patient claims that they were deprived of a genuine choice about whether to proceed or not in relation to a particular treatment. Let us assume that the duty to disclose material information set out above was breached in this case. If the case was in battery, the cause of action would have been made out. However, because the action is in negligence, the patient must still establish that the breach has caused some tangible harm.

6.5.2   To establish causation on the ordinary principles of negligence, P must demonstrate that but–for the breach they would not have suffered the harm (see Section 11.2). Therefore, the patient must be in a position to say that if they had received the warning about the risk then they would not have undergone the operation that precipitated their injury.[33] If they cannot do this then they cannot recover.[34]

6.5.3   The application of general negligence principles occurs in this area where the law is actually trying to protect the patient's interest in self-determination. This creates tension within the legal structure. An injustice can arise where P's interest in self-determination has

---

32 *Sidaway v Bethlem Royal Hospital Governors* [1985] 1 All ER 643.
33 *Smith v Tunbridge Wells* (1994) 5 Med LR 343.
34 *Smith v Barking, Havering & Brentwood Health Authority* (1994) 5 Med LR 285.

been invaded but P lacks a remedy because they cannot succeed in negligence for want of causation and/or for want of damage.[35] Faced with this question in *Chester v Afshar*,[36] the Court struggled with remaining loyal to the general principles of negligence by accepting the injustice. However, in the end, a bare majority in the House of Lords chose to depart from the rule on causation and allow recovery.[37]

Chester v Afshar [2004] UKHL 41, HL

P suffered back pain. D reviewed P and on 21 November 1994 D performed 3-level lumbar micro-discetomy. The procedure had a 1–2% inherent risk of neural damage including paralysis and *cauda equina* syndrome. This risk materialised.

At first instance it was found that: (1) D had not warned P about the risk, and so was in breach of his duty of care and (2) if the risk had been disclosed, P would have undergone the surgery but at a different date after seeking further opinions.

Held (majority decision 3:2): P could succeed.

There was sufficient legal causation between the breach of the duty to disclose and the harm suffered.

Majority (Hope Ld, Steyn Ld, Walker Ld): The very harm that it was the duty of D to warn P about has materialised. An exception to the but–for rule of causation was justified on policy grounds and to prevent the doctor's duty to disclose the risks inherent in an operation from being drained of its force. P could recover damages for the resulting harm.

Dissent (Bingham Ld, Hoffman Ld): The but–for test for causation (*see* Section 11.2) was not satisfied. It was unjust to permit recovery where the risk of harm would have been taken whether the disclosure would have been made or not.

6.5.4   The consequence is that where there is a breach of the duty to disclose and P suffers the actual harm they should have been warned about, then a claim for damages is more likely to succeed. The patient can recover if they would have deferred the procedure. They no longer

---

35   *Chappel v Hart* [1998] HCA 55, Australia High Ct www.austlii.edu.au/au/cases/cth/HCA/1998/55.html

36   [2004] UKHL 41, HL.

37   Devany, S. Autonomy rules OK. *Med Law Rev.* 2005; 13(1): 102–115.

have to demonstrate that they would have refused the procedure completely if they had been aware of the undisclosed risk.

6.5.5   The magnitude of the disclosed risk is relevant to whether it is disclosed or not but it is not the whole story. For an indication of the magnitude of risks present in the leading cases, *see* **Table 2**.

TABLE 2 Magnitude and character of risk not disclosed in the leading cases.

Case	Treatment	Risk not disclosed	Magnitude of risk	Outcome
Bolam	ECT	Acetabular fracture	1 in 50 000	Non-negligent
Rogers v Whittaker	Surgery right eye	Sympathetic ophthalmia left eye with blindness	1 in 14 000	Negligent
Sidaway	Spinal surgery	Spinal cord damage	1 in 100	Action unsuccessful
Chester v Afshar	Spinal surgery	Cauda equina syndrome	1–2 in 100	Negligent
Reibl v Hughes (Aust)	Carotid endarterectomy	Right hemiplegia	1 in 10	Negligent

6.6   CONCLUSION AND COMMENT

6.6.1   There is an elegance to a legal structure that requires doctors to owe a 'single comprehensive duty'[38] in negligence covering diagnosis and treatment, and the associated obligations to inform. Diagnosis and treatment are essentially the exercise of the medical professional skills and therefore fall fairly into the arms of negligence.

6.6.2   The duty to inform, however, seeks to protect the patient interest in self-determination.[39,40] This seems more fairly addressed by an action that is complete with the injury to the interest protected. Such an action would be more akin to an action in battery.

6.6.3   The fact that legal action for inadvertent misinformation in relation to the inherent risks/benefits of treatment lies in negligence rather than in battery leaves a legal structure that has some tension within in it.

---

38   *Sidaway v Bethlem Royal Hospital Governors* [1985] 1 All ER 643.

39   *Rogers v Whitaker* [1992] HCA 58 per Gaudron J.

40   The weakening of the causation rule in *Fairchild* (*see* Section 11.6.2) arose because causation was simply unprovable. Without the weakening of that rule injustice would have arisen. For negligent misinformation, the basis for weakening the causation rule rests on the injustice flowing from the presence of an otherwise unprotected patient interest in self-determination.

Where battery, constrained as it is by touching, is an ill-fitting robe negligence barely covers the mischief.

6.6.4 In English law negligence actions for negligent misinformation have seen this tension expressed as a strong dissent by Lord Scarmen in the case of *Sidaway v Bethlem Royal Hospital Governors*,[41] and then as a weakening of the causation rule in *Chester v Afshar*.[42,43] Notice how weakening the causation requirement makes the action of negligence more akin to a battery action – the very action precluded by the rule in *Reibl v Hughes*[44] in such cases.

6.6.5 In *Chester v Afshar* P would have had the operation at a different time and so something would have changed had the information about risk been given. The acid test of the principle in this case comes when P does not change anything as a result of the misinformation. Can they still succeed where they suffer the very harm they should have been warned about? If so, we have a negligence action that looks suspiciously like a battery action but protects the interest of self-determination.

6.6.6 The use of negligence in this context has arisen by default. The structure of a claim in negligence is simply the wrong one to protect a fundamental interest like self-determination and the strain is telling.

6.6.7 Another view is taken by Sarah Green who has pointed out that *Chester v Afshar* could be formulated as a loss of chance case (*see* Section 11.3) and in that formulation should not succeed.[45]

---

41   [1985] 1 All ER 643.
42   [2004] UKHL 41.
43   Stauch M. Taking the Consequences for failure to warn of medical risks. *Modern Law Rev.* 2000; **63**: 261.
44   (1980) 114 DLR (3d) 1, Can Sup Ct (*see* Section 6.4.2).
45   Green S. Coherence of medical negligence cases. A game of doctors and purses. *Med Law Rev.* 2006; **14**(1): 1–21.

7 Best interests

7.1.1 The best interests test operates in relation to incompetent patients. It has no relevance to decisions made by competent patients.[1]

7.1.2 The final arbiter of where the best interests of the patient lies is the Court.[2,3,4]

> 'It is, I think, important that there should not be a belief that what the doctor says is the patient's best interest *is* the patient's best interest. For my part I would certainly reserve to the court the ultimate power and duty to review the doctors' decision in the light of all the facts.'[5]

7.1.3 The Court must exercise its own judgment in light of the evidence.[6] It must consider not just the medical facts but also social, emotional, moral and welfare issues (*see* Section 7.1.9 *et seq.*).

7.1.4 Where the best interests test and the *Bolam* test reach differing conclusions it is the Court's opinion of best interest that prevails, e.g. *Re: T (a minor) (wardship: medical treatment)*[7] (*see* Section 5.5.11). Logically this means that there is only one solution to the best interests test.[8] This conclusion has consequences.

7.1.5 At common law a medical professional is bound to act within the bounds of the *Bolam* standard as modified by *Bolitho* (*see* Section 10.4).[9] Within this sphere of action they are also bound to act in the best interests of the patient.

7.1.6 Because the best interests test should give only one result, unlike the *Bolam* test which may give more than one permissible option,[10,11] there

---

1 *R v The General Medical Council* ex parte *Burke* [2004] EWHC 1879, CA.
2 *Frenchay NHS Trust v S* [1994] 2 All ER 403, 411–2 per Sir Thomas Bingham.
3 *Re: MB* (1997) 8 Med LR 217, 25 per Butler-Sloss LJ.
4 *Re: LC (medical treatment: sterilisation)* [1993] [1997] 2 FLR 258 where sterilisation was not permitted in a mentally handicapped girl because she was in a well supervised environment where the risk of pregnancy was low.
5 *Frenchay NHS Trust v S* [1994] 2 All ER 403, 411 per Sir Thomas Bingham MR.
6 *NHS Trust v A* [2005] EWCA Civ 1145, CA Section 94 per Mummery LJ.
7 [1997] 1 All ER 906.
8 *Re: S (adult patient: sterilisation)* [2001] Fam 15, 27 per Butler-Sloss P.
9 *F v West Berkshire Health Authority* [1989] 2 All ER 545, HL.
10 *Re: S (medical treatment: adult sterilisation)* [1998] 1 FLR 944.
11 *Re: S (sterilisation: patient's best interests)* [2000] 2 FLR 389.

are two duties, not one.[12] The problem with this view is that it leaves a 'Schrödinger's cat' situation. The multiple alternatives of *Bolam* must collapse to the single point of best interests, but only when the Court takes the time to open the box.[13] Thus there is an inherent ambiguity in the situation faced by medical professionals who seek to comply with the *Bolam* standard.

7.1.7   In relation to incompetent adults (including children aged 16 years and above) the *Mental Capacity Act 2005* introduces a number of additional procedures that must be attended to before a conclusion can be drawn about best interests. These include, as far as is reasonably practicable, procedures to:

(i)   Encourage and permit the person to participate in the decision-making process.[14]

(ii)   Ascertain the person's past and present wishes and feelings, their material beliefs and values, and any other factors that the person might consider if they were able to do so.[15]

(iii) Take into account and, if possible, consult:

a)   people that are engaged in caring for the person or interested in the person's welfare

b)   anyone who the person has named to be consulted, including donees of lasting powers of attorney, and

c)   any deputy appointed by the Court.[16]

7.1.8   In essence, the assessment is a balancing exercise.[17] One useful approach to determining best interests is to draw up a balance-sheet setting out the benefits and non-benefits of a proposed course of action in separate columns.[18] This was the approach used in the next case.

---

12   *Re: A (medical treatment: male sterilisation)* [2000] 1 FCR 193, 199–200 per Butler-Sloss P.
13   There is no need to separate the *Bolam* test from the best interests test for the Court: *NHS Trust v A* [2005] EWCA Civ 1145, CA para. 98 per Mummery LJ. The Court only addresses the *Bolam* test.
14   s 4(4) *Mental Capacity Act 2005.*
15   s 4(6) *Mental Capacity Act 2005.*
16   s 4(7) *Mental Capacity Act 2005.*
17   *Re: L (a minor)* [2004] EWHC 2713, paras. 12–13 per Butler-Sloss P.
18   *Re: A (medical treatment: male sterilisation)* [2000] 1 FCR 193, 205 per Thorpe LJ.

Re: A (medical treatment: male sterilisation) [2000] 1 FCR 193, CA

P was 28 years old and had Down's syndrome. He lacked capacity. He was closely supervised by his 63-year-old mother. There was concern about the consequences of any sexual activity. P was unaware of the connection between sexual activity and pregnancy.

P's mother applied for a declaration that non-therapeutic sterilisation of P would be in his best interests.

Held: Non-therapeutic sterilisation would not be in P's best interests on the present facts.

In P's current regime his level of freedom would by unaffected by sterilisation. In essence his life would be unchanged. Unlike females,[19,20,21,22] P would not suffer any risk from pregnancy nor would social disapproval of his conduct impinge upon him significantly.

7.1.9   The Court takes into account not just the medical interests of the patient but also social, emotional and other welfare issues.[23,24] Therefore, where an incompetent adult would benefit socially from the continuing welfare of a sibling, this benefit could offset the physical costs of bone marrow donation.[25]

Re: Y (adult patient) (transplant: bone marrow) [1996] 2 FLR 787, Fam

P was 36 years old and had myelodysplasia with evidence that it was transforming into acute myeloid leukaemia. P would benefit from bone marrow transplantation.

Y was P's sister. Y was a 25-year-old woman who had severe mental and physical disability together with epilepsy. She had lived in care since the age of 10 years. Y benefited from visits paid to her by P and her mother. She also benefited from occasional involvement in family events, e.g. a wedding.

Y was incompetent to consent. The risk to Y of bone marrow donation was 1 in 10 000 of death.

19   *Re: M (a minor) (wardship: sterilisation)* [1988] 2 FLR 497.
20   *Re: B (a minor) (wardship: sterilisation)* [1987] 2 All ER 206.
21   *Re: W (an adult: sterilization)* [1993] 2 FCR 187.
22   *Re: X (adult patient: sterilisation)* [1999] 3 FCR 426.
23   *Re: A (medical treatment: male sterilisation)* [2000] 1 FCR 193, 199–200 per Butler-Sloss P.
24   *Re: Y (Adult Patient) (Transplant: Bone Marrow)* [1996] 2 FLR 787.
25   *Re: Y (Adult Patient) (Transplant: Bone Marrow)* [1996] 2 FLR 787.

P applied for a declaration that it would be lawful for Y to undergo testing and possibly donate bone marrow to P.

Held: It would be lawful for Y to donate bone marrow to P as it would be to Y's emotional, psychological and social benefit.

If P died Y would loose P's visits. Also her mother would be impacted by the death. Y's relationship with her mother would be likely to suffer as P's mother would have to look after P's child. If donation occurred Y's relationship with P and her mother would be improved.

Further similar cases should be ventilated in court.

7.1.10　When this analysis does not assess it to be in the best interests of the incompetent donor to proceed with the donation then the donation will not be lawful[26] (*see* also Section 5.5.12 and 18.10.10).

Curran v Bosze (1990) 566 NE 2d 1319 (Illinois Sup Ct.)

D was the mother of 3½-year-old twins. P was the estranged father of the twins. P had a 12-year-old son from a previous marriage who was now suffering from an undifferentiated acute leukaemia. This child required bone marrow transplant.

P sought to require D to have the twins tested for compatibility with a view to bone marrow donation for the benefit of the child suffering leukaemia. D opposed the application.

Held: Testing should not proceed.

On the facts there was no social relationship between the recipient and the donors, the twins would not benefit from any bone marrow donation.

7.1.11　In certain situations the question of best interests is subject to particularly close scrutiny and an application to the Court is necessary. Two such situations are:[27]

> (i) withdrawal of artificial hydration and nutrition in cases of persistent vegetative state (*see* Section 19.10), and

---

26　*See* also *Bonner v Moran* (1941) 126 F 2d 121, USCA DC.
27　*Practice Direction (declaratory proceedings: incapacitated adults)* [2002] 1 All ER 793.

(ii) non-therapeutic sterilisation in incompetent patients. This will not be considered further here but the general principles apply.[28,29,30,31,32]

7.1.12　There is a third group of cases where it is contemplated that it would be in the best interests of an incompetent patient to make a tissue or organ donation. Obtaining the view of the Court in relation to the merits of the removal of the tissue or organ should also be considered in these cases (*see* also Section 18.10.10).[33]

7.1.13　There is a distinction between regenerative and non-regenerative organs. In the United States this reasoning has been applied to the donation of non-regenerative tissues particularly kidneys[34,35,36] (*see* also Section 18.10). This is now addressed in the UK by the *Human Tissue Act 2004* (*see* Section 18).

7.1.14　Where there is irreconcilable dispute between medical professionals, or between the medical professionals and the patient or the patient's proxy, in relation to where the patient's best interests lie, then an application to the Court is merited[37] (*see* Section 5.5.3).

7.1.15　Where the Court does determine where the best interests of the patient lie, conflict might arise where a medical professional disagrees with the opinion of the Court. The Court is very sensitive to the practical reality that delivery of care is undertaken by the responsible medical professional. The general principle is that the Court will generally not force D to treat a patient against their *bona fide* clinical judgement.

28　*Re: A (medical treatment: male sterilisation)* [2000] 1 FCR 193, 205 per Thorpe LJ.
29　*Re: M (a minor) (wardship: sterilisation)* [1988] 2 FLR 497.
30　*Re: B (a minor) (wardship: sterilisation)* [1987] 2 All ER 206.
31　*Re: W (an adult: sterilization)* [1993] 2 FCR 187.
32　*Re: X (adult patient: sterilisation)* [1999] 3 FCR 426.
33　*Re: Y (adult patient) (transplant: bone marrow)* [1996] 2 FLR 787.
34　Incompetent adult kidney donation lawful: *Strunk v Strunk* (1969) 445 SW 2d 145, Ky CA.
35　Incompetent adult permission for kidney donation refused in *Re: Guardianship of Pescinski* (1975) 226 NW 2d 180, Wisconsin Sup Ct.
36　Incompetent child kidney donation lawful: *Hart v Brown* (1972) 289 A 2d 386; in *Re: Richardson* (1973) 284 So 2d 185, Louisiana App; *Little v Little* (1979) 576 SW 2d 493, Tex Civ.
37　*R v Portsmouth Hospitals NHS Trust* ex parte *Glass* [1999] EWCA Civ 1914, CA.

Re: J (a minor)(wardship: medical treatment) [1992] 4 All ER 614,CA

Ld Donaldson MR, Balcombe, Legatt LJJ

P was a 16-month-old boy suffering microcephaly after a previous traumatic head injury received when he was one month old. He was profoundly handicapped including cortical blindness, severe cerebral palsy and epilepsy. He was fed naso-gastrically. He had made no developmental progress since the age of 10½ months. He was in the care of foster parents.

Medical evidence was that he would not develop beyond his current level. It was likely that he would deteriorate in the near future with the expectation of a short life-span. There was a risk of respiratory arrest because of the combination of the NG tube and respiratory secretions. The issue was ventilation in the event of respiratory arrest. The medical team felt it would not be appropriate to resuscitate. P's representative (the Guardian *ad litem*) favoured a DNAR order. P's mother wanted P's life preserved.

At first instance the doctors were ordered to provide ventilation and other life-sustaining treatment, including cardiopulmonary resuscitation if necessary.

Held: First instance decision reversed. It was lawful to withhold ventilation and other life-sustaining treatment.

Ld Donaldson MR

'The fundamental issue in this appeal is that whether the Court in the exercise of its inherent power to protect the interests of minors should ever require a medical practitioner or health authority acting by a medical practitioner to adopt a course of treatment which in the bona fide clinical judgement of the practitioner concerned is contraindicated as not being in the best interests of the patient.

'I cannot at present conceive of any circumstances in which this would be other than an abuse of power as directly or indirectly requiring the (medical) practitioner to act contrary to the fundamental duty which he owes to his patient.'

7.1.16   Ld Donaldson's view was supported by the entire Court. However his view is subject to the duty the Court has to protect the best interests of the child. If required to exercise the power to require treatment in the best interests of a child or an incompetent adult the Court will consider the views of the medical professionals involved.

7.1.17　If a medical professional disagrees with the Court's view of where the best interests of the patient lie then they have an obligation to offer the patient another medical opinion. This view was upheld in *Burke v GMC* (*see* Section 3.1.10).[38]

38　Contrast this with *Sawatzky v Riverview Health Centre Inc.* (1998) 167 DLR. (4th) 359.

8 Negligence: introduction

8.1 INTRODUCTION

8.1.1 Currently in NHS hospitals an NHS employer employs medical practitioners to treat patients. The contract of service is, therefore, between the NHS employer and the medical practitioner; the patient is not a party to this contract.[1] This means that the patient cannot sue either the doctor or the NHS employer on basis of this contract.[2]

8.1.2 In order to seek a remedy for inadvertent harm caused to the patient by medical professionals working within the NHS the patient must seek other avenues of redress. One such route, now increasingly commonly chosen by patients, is an action in medical negligence.

8.1.3 The essence of negligence is that:

(i) the Court will award damages

(ii) to compensate for inadvertent harm

(iii) caused to another

(iv) where the relationship is such that the harm should not have arisen.

8.1.4 The person who has suffered harm must, therefore, petition the Court and provide evidence sufficient to satisfy the Court, on a balance of probabilities, that:

(i) The relationship between the claimant and the respondent was sufficient to create an obligation on the part of the respondent to act (or not act) in a particular way, i.e. that D owed P a legal **duty of care**

(ii) The respondent in some way breached this obligation, i.e. there was a **breach of this duty of care**

---

1   *Pfizer Corporation v Ministry of Health* [1965] 1 All ER 450,HL.
2   Where there is a contract the patient can sue upon this, e.g. *Thompson v Sheffield Fertility Clinic.* High Court of Justice, Queen's Bench Division: Hooper J.; 6 March *Med Law Rev.* 2001; 9: 170188. The mother settled for £20000 out of Court.

(iii) As a result of that breach (i.e **causation**) the claimant suffered the harm which is the basis of the complaint

(iv) This harm suffered by the claimant must be such that the Court will recognise it and will require that damages are paid by the respondent to the claimant in compensation for it, i.e. there was some consequent legally recognised **damage**.

8.1.5 These are the four core elements of negligence. Just step back briefly and notice how it is fair to ask someone (D) who has a particular responsibility arising from a particular relationship with another person (P) to conduct themselves in a way that does not cause harm to that other person (P) by failing to discharge that responsibility.

8.1.6 It will be convenient to consider the types of recognised damage in the section on duty of care (*see* Section 9). We will not consider how damages are quantified or awarded.

8.2   GROSS NEGLIGENCE

8.2.1 For negligence the harm does not need to be intended (for more on intention, *see* Section 19.6). The harm can arise through inadvertence. The purpose of negligence is to compensate where it is just to do so. It is not about punishing wrongdoing. However, if the harm was intentional or recklessly committed, then questions about punishment arise and the criminal law may be invoked. This border of criminal liability can be crossed if the negligence is gross and the harm severe. In such cases of gross negligence criminal sanctions may be merited.

R v Adomako [1994] 3 All ER 79, HL

D was an anaesthetist. During an eye operation D did not notice that the oxygen tube had disconnected from the ventilator for six minutes. As a result P suffered a cardiac arrest and subsequently died.

D was convicted of manslaughter in the Crown court by a jury majority verdict of 11:1. D appealed.

Held: Conviction for involuntary manslaughter by breach of duty (gross negligence) upheld.

8.3 PRIVATE HEALTHCARE

8.3.1   In relation to private healthcare the contract of service is between the patient and the doctor. A duty of care arising from the doctor–patient relationship still exists, albeit that the relationship here is created by the private contract. The private contract itself may create additional rights and duties above those present imposed by the duty of care in tort – these depend upon the terms of the agreement. It is important to note that a contract cannot be used to restrict liability for negligence, particularly in relation to physical injury or death.[3]

---

3   s 2 *Unfair Contract Terms Act 1977.*

9 Negligence: the duty of care

9.1 DUTY OF CARE

9.1.1   The idea of the duty of care is introduced in Section 8.1.4. It is important for healthcare professionals to understand to whom, and in relation to what types of harm, such duties are owed. If there is no duty of care owed by a healthcare professional to a particular person in relation to a particular type of harm, then an action of negligence cannot be maintained against that professional should that particular type of harm arise.

9.1.2   The duty of care arises from certain relationships within society. Broadly there are three main approaches to discovering if a duty of care exists in a particular situation:[1]

(i)   An incremental approach: here previous cases are examined and the duty of care arises if the duty of care exists in analogous cases. This applies in most cases (*see* Section 2.3.3)

(ii)   An assumption of responsibility: where there is an undertaking of an obligation that does not amount to a legal contract[2,3]

(iii)   A tripartite formula: this approach has been arrived at following development in a long line of legal cases.[4,5] It is a return to first principles. The three stages are:

a)   foreseeability: is it reasonably foreseeable that the act (or omission in breach of duty) complained about would have caused the harm complained about?

---

1   *BCCI v Price Waterhouse* [1998] Lloyd's Rep. Bank 85, CA per Sir Brian Neill.
2   *Hedley Byrne & Co Ltd v Heller & Partners Ltd* [1963] 2 All ER 575; *Henderson v Merrett Syndicates Ltd* [1994] 3 All ER 506 – an assumption of responsibility and reliance upon that assumption are required here; *White v Jones* [1995] 1 All ER 691.
3   *Capital Counties plc v Hampshire CC* [1997] 2 All ER 865, 883 CA.
4   *Donoghue v Stevenson* [1932] All ER Rep 1; *Hedley Byrne & Co Ltd v Heller & Partners Ltd* [1963] 2 All ER 575; *Home Office v Dorset Yacht Co Ltd* [1970] 2 All ER 294; *Anns v London Borough of Merton* [1977] 2 All ER 492; *Junior Books Ltd v Veitchi Co Ltd* [1982] 3 All ER 201; *Yuen Kun-Yeu v A-G of Hong Kong* [1987] 2 All ER 705.
5   *Caparo Industries plc v Dickman* [1990] 1 All ER 568.

b) <u>proximity</u>: is there a sufficiently close relationship between the two parties to give rise to a legal obligation to compensate for the harm complained about?

c) <u>fair, just and reasonable</u>: is it fair, just and reasonable for the injured party to receive compensation? (However, the court will also consider the impact of the existence of a duty upon all cases of that type.)[6]

9.2 DOCTOR AND PATIENT

9.2.1 A doctor–patient relationship generates a duty of care owed by the doctor to the patient.[7] Something must operate to bring two people into a doctor–patient relationship before a duty of care can be created. Usually an undertaking is necessary but this does not have to be formally expressed. It can arise from the circumstances.

Barnett v Chelsea & Kensington Hospital Management Committee [1968] 1 All ER 1068, QBD

Three watchmen attended an accident and emergency department suffering from vomiting. The doctors were made aware of their presence but the watchmen were sent home without being seen. One of the watchmen, who was suffering from arsenic poisoning, subsequently died.

Held: D not liable.

Attending the accident and emergency department was sufficient to create a duty of care owed by the Hospital and the duty doctor to the patient.

However, it was also found that even if the patient had been attended to the death could not have been prevented. The case therefore failed on causation (*see* Section 11).

9.2.2 This duty of care is owed by the doctor to the patient. The patient is the person seeking medical care. A duty of care is virtually always owed by the responsible medical professional to their patient.

---

6 Rogers WVH. *Winfield & Jolowicz on Tort*. 17th ed. London: Sweet & Maxwell; 2006. p. 135.

7 *R v Bateman* [1925] All ER Rep 45, CCA per Hewart CJ.

9.2.3   If the negligence occurs outside the NHS then only the practitioner is liable.[8,9]

9.3   DUTIES TO THIRD PARTIES

9.3.1   Duties to third parties *may* be created, for example, where an identifiable third party is at personal risk of physical harm from the patient.[10,11] But, in general, duties to third parties are not automatically created by virtue of a pre-existing doctor–patient relationship. This is so even if it is the pre-existing doctor–patient relationship that brings the doctor and the third party into close contact.

Powell v Boldaz (1997) 39 BMLR 35, CA

P was a child aged 10 years 4 months who died after failure to diagnose Addison's disease. D settled their liability to P in an out-of-court settlement for £100 000.

P's parents brought a further action alleging a 'cover-up' after the death resulting in them suffering psychiatric harm and economic loss.

Held: D owed a duty of care to P because P was seeking medical care. D did not owe a duty of care to P's parents.[12]

9.3.2   It is incorrect to assume that no duties arise from the relationship that exists between the doctor and the parents in a situation like that in *Powell v Boldaz*.[13] But the relationship between the doctor and the parents in this situation is not one of doctor and patient.

9.3.3   Healthcare professionals were not held to owe a duty of care to the parents (as third parties) for harm they suffer as a result of negligence that occurs within the doctor–patient (child) relationship.

---

8   *Ellis v Wallsend District Hospital* (1989) 17 NSWLR 533, NSW CA.
9   *Yepremian v Scarborough Hospital* (1980) 110 DLR (3d) 513, Ont CA.
10   *Tarasoff v Regents of University of California* (1976) 17 Cal 3d 425.
11   Note that in the Californian case of *Reisner v Regents of University of California* (1995) 31 Cal App 4th 1195, 37 Cal Rptr 2d 518 a non-identifiable third party who became infected with HIV from P was able to sue for D's failure to inform P that she was HIV-positive. This is perhaps best seen as foreseeable damage lying within the scope of the breach of D's duty to disclose to P.
12   For subsequent developments *see Powell v Boldaz* [2003] EWHC 2160.
13   *See* Kennedy I, Grubb A. (eds) *Principles of Medical Law*. Butterworths: 1998. para. 5.87.

JD v East Berkshire Community Health NHS Trust [2005] UKHL 23,HL[14]

Three separate cases. Doctors and social workers had suspected that children were suffering or at risk of non-accidental injury. After investigation, in each case no evidence of non-accidental injury was found. The medical conditions were: multiple severe allergies, Schamberg's disease (progressive pigmented purpuric dermatitis) and osteogenesis imperfecta.

The parents each sued the respective doctors and Hospital Trusts only in negligence.

Held (4:1): Where doctors and social workers acted on good faith in what they believed were the best interests of the child no duty of care was owed by the doctors to the parents of children simply because they were parents of the respective doctor's patient.

This was on the grounds of public policy and because it was not fair, just and reasonable to extend the duty of care to parents in this situation. When considering the possibility of non-accidental injury there was a conflict of interests between the child and the parent. In such circumstances the doctor should not be faced with potentially conflicting duties.

It is of note that the events litigated had occurred before the *Human Rights Act 1998* had come into force. Therefore, there was no claim made based upon those rights. It is possible that a claim based upon the new rights may be successful.[15]

9.3.4   Other examples where a close relationship between a doctor and another person does not create a doctor–patient relationship include (i) communicating to others about a patient and (ii) assessing a person on behalf of someone else.[16]

9.3.5   Where a doctor who has been caring for a patient that has died communicates that fact to the relatives, duties do exist but they are not based upon the doctor–patient relationship that existed between the doctor and the deceased patient.[17]

---

14   *See*, also, *Sullivan v Moody* (2001) 207 CLR 562, Australia High Ct; *B v A-G of New Zealand* [2003] 4 All ER 833, PC.

15   *See* the dissent of Bingham Ld. Rodger Ld reserved his position on this point (para. 118). *See*, also, *Z v United Kingdom* [2001] 2 FCR 246 and *TP v United Kingdom* [2001] 2 FCR 289.

16   *West Bromwich Albion Football Club Ltd v El-Safty* [2005] EWHC 2866.

17   *Powell v Boldaz* (1997) 39 BMLR 35 per Smith LJ.

9.3.6   Where a psychiatrist is retained by a local authority in order to discharge its care responsibilities and in that role the psychiatrist examines
a child and interviews a parent no doctor–patient relationship is
created.[18] The same is true by analogy where a doctor examines a
patient on behalf of an insurance company.

Baker v Kaye (1997) 39 BMLR 12

D assessed P at a pre-employment medical check. P gave a history of
35 units of alcohol per week. Blood tests revealed P to have a raised gamma
GT – 137 IU/L (NR: <60 IU/L)) and mixed hyperlipidaemia (cholesterol
9.3 mmol/L; triglycerides 5.46 mmol/L (NR 0.8–2.0 mmol/L)).

P claimed that D had made a statement to him to the effect that the
medical examination was satisfactory. On the strength of this P resigned
his current position.

D consulted with a hepatologist and notified the potential employers that
there was a risk of excessive alcohol intake. The company's culture sought to
avoid employees' consumption of alcohol where it might reflect unfavourably
upon the company. The company refused to appoint P to the job because it
involved frequent business-related socialising.

P claimed for loss of earnings (economic loss) arising from the statement
given to him by D.

Held: D not liable.

D did owe P a duty in relation to economic loss suffered by P arising out
of the medical examination where D conducted that medical examination on
behalf of a third party. However D had conducted the examination and given
the report competently. The conclusion about alcohol intake met the *Bolam*
standard, therefore D was not in breach of this duty.

9.3.7   The scope of the duty of care owed to the patient when assessing
them on behalf of a third party is limited to those harms that foresee-
ably flow from the breach and for which it is just to permit recovery
(*see* Section 9.5). Thus it was held in the next case that a missed
radiological diagnosis in the context of a pre-employment check did
not give rise to liability for the costs of bringing up a healthy child
until adulthood.

---

18   *X and others (minors) v Bedfordshire CC* [1995] 3 All ER 353, HL.

R v Croyden (1990) 40 BMLR 40, CA

P had a pre-employment interview including a CXR. A radiologist (D) failed to note pulmonary vessel enlargement. P subsequently became pregnant. Whilst pregnant P was diagnosed as having primary pulmonary hypertension (PPH).

P alleged wrongful conception (see paras. 13.2.6–13.2.12) claiming that if D had interpreted the CXR correctly then she would have been diagnosed as suffering from PPH. If P had been aware of diagnosis of PPH then she would not have undertaken pregnancy because of the risks involved.

Held: P did not recover for the costs of bringing up a healthy child because the duty owed by D to P in relation to the pregnancy was in relation to a pre-employment CXR. The possibility of pregnancy was not within the scope of this duty of care.

However the failure to diagnose was a breach of duty and, therefore, P did recover for the harm which might have been avoided if the CXR diagnosis had been made, including the complications of pregnancy attributable to PPH and invasive cardiac investigations that might have been avoided had an earlier diagnosis been made.

9.3.8　Another example might be in **rescue situations**.[19] A doctor who is simply passing the scene of an accident is not obliged in law to attend a victim of a road traffic accident purely because an emergency arises.[20,21] It should be noted, though, that whilst this is the position in law, there is a professional duty to assist in emergencies imposed by the General Medical Council.[22,23]

9.3.9　However, once a doctor intervenes they would appear to enter a doctor–patient relationship with the victim through an implied undertaking of responsibility. It is possible that, in this situation, the scope of the duty of care may only extend to not making the situation worse rather than a requirement to strive for a cure.[24]

19　*Baker v Hopkins* [1959] 1 WLR 966; *Ogwo v Taylor* [1988] AC 431.
20　*Horsley v MacLaren, The Ogopogo* [1972] SCR 441, Supreme Ct Canada.
21　*Capital and Counties v Hampshire CC* [1997] 2 All ER 865 per Stuart-Smith LJ.
22　*Good Medical Practice*. General Medical Council. 2006. para. 11.
23　Note, also, *Lowns v Woods* (1996) Aust Torts Reports; pp. 81–376 (NSWCA) and the strong dissent of Mahoney JA.
24　*Horsley v MacLaren, The Ogopogo* [1972] SCR 441, Supreme Ct Canada.

9.3.10 These principles are subject to the contractual obligation that is owed by holders of a General Medical Services Contract to people in their practice area to whom they have been requested to attend during core hours,[25,26] and by hospital practitioners to patients in their hospital.

9.4 AMBULANCES

9.4.1 Interestingly, it has been held that emergency services, including fire brigade,[27] police[28] and coastguard,[29] owe a duty to the public in general but not to particular individuals.

9.4.2 However, it seems that ambulances are not stand-alone emergency services but part of the NHS. Once an ambulance call is accepted, a duty of care exists between the ambulance service and the individual on whose behalf the ambulance was called. The duty is to arrive in a reasonable time. Conflicting priorities or a plea of resource constraints may mitigate this duty.[30]

Kent v Griffiths [2000] 2 All ER 474, CA

P suffered an asthma attack and called their GP. The GP called the London Ambulance Service (LAS) at 16:25, gave details and asked for an ambulance 'immediately please'. This call was accepted. Ambulance arrived at P's home at 17:05; P arrived at hospital at 17:17. P suffered a respiratory arrest.

Ambulance recorded time of arrival at P's home as 16:47.

First instance held if ambulance had arrived in a reasonable time then there was a high probability that P would not have suffered a respiratory arrest. No satisfactory explanation had been given for the length of time taken to arrive at the scene. Record of time of arrival had been falsified contemporaneously. In the absence of reasonable excuse, the delay was culpable.

---

25 para. 15(6) *National Health Service (General Medical Services Contracts) Regulations 2004* SI 2004/291.

26 Core hours means: 8am and ending at 6.30pm on any day from Monday to Friday except Good Friday, Christmas Day or bank holidays.

27 *Capital and Counties plc v Hampshire CC* [1997] 2 All ER 865.

28 *Hill v Chief Constable of West Yorkshire* [1988] 2 All ER 238; *Alexandrou v Oxford* [1993] 4 All ER 32. But note *Reeves v Metropolitan Police Commmisioner* [1999] 3 All ER 897.

29 *OLL Ltd v Secretary of State for Transport* [1997] 3 All ER 897.

30 For an assessment of the financial impact of this rule *see* Williams K. Litigation against English NHS ambulance services and the rule in *Kent v Griffiths. Med Law Rev.* 2007; 15(2): 153–75.

LAS appealed on the basis that they did not owe a duty of care to a member of the public upon whose behalf a 999 call was made.

Held: Duty of care existed. P was entitled to damages.

9.5 DUTY OF CARE IN RELATION TO PARTICULAR TYPES OF HARM SUFFERED

9.5.1 The physical integrity of individuals is jealously protected by the Courts. Therefore, the Courts will much more readily find a duty of care is owed where physical harm is the damage complained about. Psychiatric harm is regarded as a species of physical injury but the duty to avoid causing psychiatric injury, where it is suffered alone, is only owed to a restricted class of people. This is to avoid large numbers of claims arising in certain situations (the floodgates argument).

9.5.2 Similarly, damage to property is also granted significant protection – although this can be reduced to mere monetary loss in some situations.[31] In some cases, several different types of loss may be considered. For example, unwanted pregnancy is seen as a type of physical harm from which the costs of bringing up the child are a type of consequent financial loss (*see* also Section 13 and para. 13.2.18).

Walkin v South Manchester HA **[1995] 4 All ER 132, CA**

P sought sterilisation for financial reasons. D negligently performed sterilisation by laparoscopic tubal diathermy. P subsequently became pregnant.

P sued for negligent performance of the procedure causing wrongful conception (an action that is no longer sustainable, *see* Section 13.2.14), and failure to inform of risk of failure (*see* Section 6.5).

The claim for personal injury (i.e. the pregnancy) was barred by statute, so P claimed for recovery of her financial loss.

Held: P could not recover.

The financial loss flowed from the pregnancy thus the action was one for personal injury rather than pure financial loss. Therefore, it fell within the terms of Section 38(1) of the Limitation Act 1980 and was statute barred.

---

31   *Murphy v Brentwood DC* [1990] 2 All ER 908.

9.6 PSYCHIATRIC HARM

9.6.1 Psychiatric harm must be sufficiently severe to be recognised as a psychiatric illness.[32,33] Here, there is a distinction between primary and secondary victims:

(i) *Primary victims* are those where the psychiatric harm arises in a situation where the victim suffers physical harm or could have suffered physical harm from the negligence

(ii) *Secondary victims* are those where the victim suffers the psychiatric harm by apprehending others who have suffered harm from the negligence, i.e. there was no direct physical threat to the person suffering the psychiatric harm.[34]

9.6.2 For primary victims, the situation is akin to recovering for physical harm.[35] For secondary victims, constraints apply to restrict those who can recover from the negligent person, in which situations and the extent to which they can recover.

9.6.3 **Primary victims:**[36] When physical harm is suffered as a result of the negligence then the connected psychiatric injury, as a species of physical injury, is generally recoverable. Therefore, a duty of care is owed in relation to psychiatric harm suffered in this way.

9.6.4 Where physical injury could have resulted but only psychiatric harm did in fact result, then the psychiatric harm is recoverable on the same basis as the physical injury. Such psychiatric harm may be suffered because the injured person was personally at risk from the danger created by the negligent act or omission.[37]

9.6.5 Because this is regarded as a type of physical harm similarly generous rules apply to what can be recovered for the psychiatric harm as apply to physical injury. For example, the 'eggshell skull' principle applies whereby the victim must be accepted with whatever natural vulnerabilities they possess.

---

32 *Hinz v Berry* [1970] 1 All ER 1074 where this was clinical depression.
33 *Younger v Dorset and Somerset Strategic HA* [2006] Lloyd's Rep Med 489.
34 *Bourhill v Young* [1942] UKHL 5.
35 *Page v Smith* [1995] 2 All ER 736, 766 per Ld Lloyd.
36 *Page v Smith* [1995] 2 All ER 736, 766 per Ld Lloyd.
37 *Chadwick v British Transport Commission* [1967] 2 All ER 945 – anxiety neurosis after assisting at the scene of the Lewisham rail disaster in 1957.

Page v Smith [1995] 2 All ER 736, HL

P had suffered myalgic encephalomyelitis (ME) for 20 years and was in remission. P was involved, but physically unhurt, in a road accident caused by the negligence of D. As a result of the accident P's ME relapsed.

P claimed damages in negligence for the nervous shock and consequent relapse of his ME.

At first instance: P recovered £162 153.

Court of Appeal: The decision was reversed. D argued that the relapse of the ME was not a foreseeable consequence of the road accident.

Held: P could recover on the basis of an 'eggshell personality' (see para. 9.6.5).

A further issue relating to causation was returned to the Court of Appeal for consideration.

9.6.6　　Despite this rule, the court will not allow recovery in every instance. In the next case, note also the length of time between the negligence, the initiation of the legal action and its final resolution. (For a fuller discussion of the law of surrogacy see Section 16.)

Briody v St. Helen's & Knowsley Area Health Authority [2001] EWCA Civ 1010, CA

P was 19 years old. A year earlier she had suffered a traumatic stillbirth requiring emergency section. She had become pregnant again and was in hospital for the birth. She became acutely unwell during labour and underwent emergency surgery. This revealed a rupture at the site of the uterine scar necessitating sub-total hysterectomy but with ovarian preservation. Sadly, this child was also stillborn.

19 years later P sued for negligence. Because of legal delays (nine further years), by the time the case eventually came to the Court of Appeal P was 47 years old.

Negligence was conceded and P succeeded in recovering damages for pain and suffering, and for loss of amenity. P made further claims including those for:

(i) psychiatric injury as a primary victim (see Section 9.6.1), and

(ii) the costs of surrogacy treatment. There were two possible options for the surrogacy agreement:

a) using P's eggs and her partner's sperm, or

b) donor eggs and her partner's sperm.

The preferred option was (a) and the plan was to have it carried out in California under a binding surrogacy agreement governed by Californian law. (Another option involving a surrogacy arrangement in the UK to be governed by English law was putative.)

Initial medical evidence was that the probability of a successful pregnancy using a surrogate mother depended on the age of the mother's eggs: 45 years – 1.5%, 46 years – 2.4%, 47 years – 0%, 48 years – 0%. With donor eggs, the chances of success were estimated at up to 25% per cycle.

Surrogacy per se was not illegal, although a contract for surrogacy was unenforceable in English law.

At first instance: P's claim for psychiatric injury was successful. P recovered some £66000. Her claim for the costs of the surrogacy treatment failed.

P appealed against the latter decision, introducing fresh evidence on appeal. Six embryos had been created using P's eggs and P's partner's sperm. The medical evidence was that the chance of a successful pregnancy had increased to 1% by virtue of this fact.

P now preferred the option of a surrogate arrangement in the UK arranged through COTS[38] with the agreement covered by English law. The putative plan was for two cycles with embryos created using P's eggs; if unsuccessful, then four cycles with the surrogate's eggs with the option of three further cycles to have a second child.

Held CA: P could not recover for the costs of the surrogacy.

Because it was not illegal, in principle recovery for the costs of surrogacy as damages in a civil legal action was not precluded on public policy grounds.

The chances of a successful pregnancy in a surrogate mother using P's own eggs were remote even after the creation of the embryos.

It was not reasonable to ask the defendant to pay for a treatment that would be unlikely to succeed. Nor was it reasonable to ask the defendant to pay for a treatment that did not return P to the position she would have been in had the negligence not occurred.

The chances of success with donor eggs was high. However, with donor eggs neither the eggs nor the pregnancy belonged to P. The situation was akin to adoption.

---

38 Childlessness Overcome Through Surrogacy.

What P had lost through the negligence was the ability to have a pregnancy. The chance to have genetically-related children was lost by passage of time. The delay was the fault of neither party.

What P had lost, the chance to have a pregnancy, could not be recovered and must be compensated for within the damages she had received for pain, suffering and loss of amenity including the award for psychiatric harm.

She had no right to be provided with a child even under Article 12 of the European Convention of Human Rights: the right to marry and found a family.

9.6.7   There is a duty to not disclose bad news to patients in a way that might cause psychiatric harm.

AB v Tameside & Glossop HA (1997) 8 Med LR 91, CA

The fact that an obstetric healthcare worker was found to be HIV-positive was pre-emptively disclosed to the public by the media. The Hospital had been in the process of making arrangements for patients who had been in contact with the worker to be notified by post of the diagnosis.

An action was brought by patients of the Hospital to recover damages for psychiatric harm, claiming that the information should have been transmitted face to face rather than by letter.

Held: The patients could not recover because the Hospital had taken reasonable steps to ensure that the news was broken appropriately. However, a duty of care did exist in relation to the way in which this type of bad news was broken.

Natural distress alone would not amount to psychiatric injury or illness.[39]

9.6.8   When the bad news given to a patient is incorrect, the patient may recover for psychiatric injury.

Allin v City and Hackney Health Authority (1996) 7 Med LR 167

A 30-year-old mother had a very difficult birth involving *vasa previa* and haemorrhage. The child had no discernable heartbeat for 22 minutes after

---

39   *AB v Tameside & Glossop HA* (1997) 8 Med LR 91, 99 per Brooke LJ.

delivery. The mother was told after this that her child had not survived.

In fact the baby had survived and was attending school at the time of the trial. The mother only learnt of the survival of her child when one of the doctors spoke of the child using the present tense.

Held: The mother could recover for psychiatric injury (post traumatic stress disorder) that resulted from receiving the misinformation.

9.6.9   Notice how the harm in relation to disclosing information to patients appears to fall under the heading of primary liability for psychiatric harm. Because of this, the particular vulnerabilities of the patient are relevant – at least to the extent of the damages that can be recovered. This result may arise because the harm arises in the context of the doctor–patient relationship and there is a duty to avoid causing harm within that relationship.

9.6.10   **Secondary victims:**[40] It is conceivable that anyone watching, for example, a cardiac arrest being treated, could suffer psychiatric harm. In some cases damages can be recovered for this psychiatric harm. Because the potential size of the group of people who might claim is so large and the extent of the potential liability so great, the Courts have constrained both the size of the group to whom a duty of care is owed in this way and the extent of the duty owed.

9.6.11   There are conditions on the group of people to whom this duty is owed:

(i)   the secondary victim must have a close relationship of love and affection with the primary victim of the negligence

(ii)   the psychiatric harm suffered by the secondary victim must be caused by the direct perception of the accident or its direct aftermath, and

(iii)   the secondary victim must have been present at the accident or immediate aftermath.

9.6.12   Recovery was permitted in the next case.[41]

---

40   *McLoughlin v O'Brian* [1982] 2 All ER 298.
41   *See*, also, *North Glamorgan NHS Trust v Walters* [2002] EWCA Civ 1792.

McLoughlin v O'Brian [1982] 2 All ER 298, HL

P's husband and three children were involved in a road traffic accident caused by D's negligence. One child was killed, the other two children were severely injured and her husband was hurt. P discovered what had happened one hour later and immediately went to the hospital. There she saw the injuries her family suffered.

As a result of this experience she suffered organic depression and other psychological symptoms.

Held: P could recover for her psychiatric harm.

9.6.13   But recovery was not permitted when the all the criteria in Section 9.6.11 were not met. For example where the secondary victims either: did not perceive the accident or its aftermath directly; or were not present at the scene of the accident.

Alcock v Chief Constable of the South Yorkshire Police [1991] 4 All ER 907, HL

Hillsborough disaster. Police negligently allowed excessively large numbers of people into an already full football stadium. 95 people were crushed to death and 400 people were injured.

16 relatives of disaster victims, some who were at the match but not at the actual scene of the disaster, sought to claim for psychiatric harm (nervous shock).

Held: None of the relatives could recover.

9.6.14   Some of the police officers at the Hillsborough disaster were also affected by the scenes, suffering post-traumatic stress disorder as a result.[42] They were not primary victims. They were unsuccessful in their action for compensation for psychiatric harm as secondary victims on similar grounds to those set out in Section 9.6.13, i.e. despite being rescuers they lacked a close relationship of love and affection with the victims. It also seemed unjust to permit them to

---

42   *White v Chief Constable of the South Yorkshire Police* [1998] UKHL 45; [1999] 1 All ER 1.

recover damages when the close relatives had been turned away with empty hands in *Alcock v Chief Constable of the South Yorkshire Police*.[43]

9.6.15   The extent of the duty owed to secondary victims is also constrained. For example, the 'eggshell skull' rule (*see* para. 9.6.5) does not operate.[44] Thus, the duty is only owed to the extent of foreseeable psychiatric harm to people with ordinary phleghm.[45]

9.7   FINANCIAL HARM

9.7.1   This is economic loss, i.e. the loss of money or the failure to acquire money or its equivalent. If the financial loss arises because of physical injury then it can be recovered. One example might be earnings lost through sickness caused by another's negligence. But financial losses unconnected to the physical injury itself are not recoverable, except in certain situations.[46]

9.7.2   Financial losses unconnected to the physical injury itself are recoverable when:

   (i)   a patient seeks the advice of a medical professional

   (ii) for a purpose that could result in monetary loss to the patient, and

   (iii) the medical professional is aware of that purpose and

   (iv) gives advice that is negligent, and

   (v)   the patient acts in reliance upon the medical advice, and suffers monetary loss because of that reliance.

Only if all of the above criteria are met may patient recover for the monetary loss flowing from the negligent advice.[47]

9.7.3   If the medical professional is not aware of the purpose in this context, or the patient relies upon the information for some other purpose, then the patient may not recover for monetary loss.[48]

---

43   [1991] 4 All ER 907.
44   *Page v Smith* [1995] 2 All ER 736, 766 per Ld Lloyd.
45   *Bourhill v Young* [1942] UKHL 5, per Porter Ld at para. 44.
46   *Spartan Steel and Alloys Ltd v Martin & Co (Contractors) Ltd* [1972] 3 All ER 557.
47   *Hedley Byrne & Co Ltd v Heller & Partners Ltd* [1963] 2 All ER 575.
48   *Caparo Industries plc v Dickman* [1990] 1 All ER 568.

Stevens v Bermondsey and Southwark Group HMC (1963) 107 SJ 478

After an accident P was advised by a casualty doctor that nothing was wrong. In reliance on D's statement P settled his accident claim. P subsequently developed spinal spondylosis. P sued D for economic loss flowing from the negligent misstatement.

Held: No duty was owed by D in relation to financial events; a duty was only owed in relation to physical harm.

9.7.4   In *Baker v Kaye*[49] (*see* Section 9.3.6), the combination of a claim for financial loss and the fact that the doctor was examining P on behalf of a third party (i.e. there was no doctor–patient relationship) made it hard for P to recover.[50]

9.7.5   If references are not diligently completed[51] the employee may recover the economic losses resulting from a negligently prepared reference.

Spring v Guardian Assurance PLC [1994] 3 All ER 129, HL

P was dismissed by his employer, D. P applied for another job with another company (C). C sought a reference from D. The reference was unfavourable and P was not appointed by C.
    P sued the defendants for negligent preparation of the reference.

Held: P recovered for his economic loss resulting from the negligently prepared employment reference.

9.7.6   The GMC has issued guidance on the writing of references.[52]

9.8   DUTY OF CARE OWED BY NHS HOSPITALS TO PATIENTS

9.8.1   The key thing to remember is that the NHS Trust is a distinct legal entity. Thus there are three parties in the relationship – the NHS Trust, the employees of the NHS Trust and the patient.

---

49   (1997) 39 BMLR 12.
50   *See*, also, *West Bromwich Albion Football Club Ltd v El-Safty* [2005] EWHC 2866.
51   *Hassan v Sandwell & West Birmingham Hospital NHS Trust* [2006] EWHC 2407.
52   GMC guidance. Writing References. 8 August 2007. *See* www.gmc-uk.org/guidance/.

9.8.2   There are two main ways in which NHS Trusts might owe a duty of care to a patient: directly or indirectly.

9.8.3   The indirect duty comes in two flavours – vicarious and non-delegable. In practice, the most important duty by far is the indirect duty of vicarious liability. (*See* also **Figure 1**, p. 136 and **Figure 2**, p. 139.) We will not consider the somewhat rarefied concept of the indirect non-delegable duty of care here.

9.8.4   **Vicarious liability:**[53,54] This arises on the basis that an employer is responsible for the actions of its employees. The Hospital is responsible to the patient for the negligence of its employees if the negligence occurred during the course of the employment of that employee.

9.8.5   The medical professional remains liable for the negligence but, because the medical professional is placed in the relationship as a result of a contract of service with the NHS employer, the NHS employer is also held liable for the negligence. The claimant can choose to sue either or both parties – but often chooses to sue the NHS Trust because it is usually covered by the NHS medical indemnity scheme.[55]

9.8.6   **Direct duty of care:** This is owed by the Hospital to the patient whereby it is directly responsible to the patient for its own negligence. For example, the Hospital is obliged to ensure that the systems for the provision of care to the patient are such that as might be reasonably expected of a hospital of that size and type.[56] There is also a statutory responsibility to ensure and improve the quality of services provided.[57]

---

53 *Gold v Essex County Council* [1942] 2 All ER 237 – radiographer, negligent radiation treatment.
54 *Cassidy v Ministry of Health* [1951] 1 All ER 574 – negligent surgery for Dupytren's contracture.
55 The Clinical Negligence Scheme for Trusts. Created by the *NHS (Clinical Negligence Scheme) Regulations 1996* (SI 1996/251).
56 *See*, also, *Cassidy v Ministry of Health* [1951] 1 All ER 574, *Jones v Manchester Corporation* [1952] 2 All ER 125; *Roe v Minister of Health* [1954] 2 All ER 13; *Wilsher v Essex AHA* [1986] 3 All ER 801, 830, 832 CA; *X (minors) v Bedfordshire County Council* [1995] 3 All ER 353, 371 per Ld Browne-Wilkinson. In Australia a similar duty has been recognised: *Ellis v Wallsend District Hospital* (1989) 17 NSWLR 533, NSW CA whilst in Canada no non-delegable duty was found: *Yepremian v Scarborough Hospital* (1980) 110 DLR (3d) 513, Ont CA.
57 s 18 *Health Act 1999*.

Bull v Devon AHA (1993) 4 Med LR 117, CA

The Hospital provided an obstetric service on one site, with the gynaecological service offered at another site one mile away. P delivered monozygotic twins after 33 weeks of pregnancy. The first child was delivered but there were difficulties with the delivery of the second twin, who was in the breech position, including bleeding suggesting *abruptio placenta*. There was a delay in obtaining the attendance of a suitably qualified doctor.

The second twin was born 68 minutes after the first twin and suffered hypoxic brain injury. He suffered severe mental disability and quadriplegia.

The action was brought 17 years after the event.

Held: The Hospital was negligent in failing to provide in a timely fashion the skilled care P had required.

The failure arose because there was an inefficient system for calling the doctor. It was possible for the delay to have occurred without negligence on the part of any individual, rather simply as a result of the way the system was ordered. The unexplained nature of the delay required the Hospital to justify it,[58] but this they had failed to do.[59]

9.8.7   More specifically, the duties are to: provide access to hospital care; provide appropriate staff and facilities; ensure that treatment is administrated with adequate care; and an obligation to ensure that the correct care is delivered.[60]

Robertson (an infant) v Nottingham Health Authority (1997) 8 Med LR 1,[61] CA

Baby Jessica suffered multicystic-leuco-encephalo-malacia ('MCLE') with consequent severe spastic quadriplegia, epilepsy, mental and visual impairment, and microcephaly. Prior to delivery she had developed cardiac decelerations. The first cardiotocogram ('CTG') trace was normal. Communication breakdowns lead to more CTGs than necessary before a caesarean was performed. Caesarean section was performed after the seventh CTG trace, with a maximum unjustified delay of two hours.

---

58   *Richards v Swansea NHS Trust* [2007] EWHC 487.
59   The evidential burden of proof had shifted by virtue of the *res ipsa loquitur* doctrine.
60   *A (a child) v Ministry of Defence* [2004] EWCA 641, para. 32 per Ld Phillips MR.
61   Also known as *Re: R (a minor) (No. 2)* (1997) 33 BMLR 178.

The baby was delivered in a poor state – APGAR score of 4 – and suffered seizures post-delivery.

Held CA: There was a direct duty of care owed by a hospital to a patient. That duty was to establish a proper system of care such as can be reasonably expected of a hospital of that size and type.

P's claim was unsuccessful, despite the presence of negligence, because the negligence did not cause the harm complained about. The delay in the caesarean section was negligent but the cerebral damage was not due to the acute hypoxic injury, rather to a non-negligent chronic prenatal hypoxic insult.

9.8.8 One old case[62] addresses the question of which duty was applicable: either the duty owed by the doctor to the patient, or the duty owed by the Hospital to the patient. This fact underlines the importance of vicarious liability in the context of the modern situation. In that case, the patient died from an ill-administered anaesthetic. The Hospital sought an indemnity for the legal action from the doctor. They failed because they had contributed to the harm by permitting an inexperienced doctor to deliver an anaesthetic without supervision.

9.8.9 In the more recent case of *Garcia v St. Mary's NHS Trust*,[63] bleeding after coronary bypass graft surgery led to brain injury. The surgery was found not to have been negligently performed. However there was a gap of 31 minutes from the time of the crash call to the arrival of the cardiothoracic registrar who eventually controlled the bleeding by re-opening the patient. The Court (albeit at first instance) found a duty of care was owed by the Trust directly to the patient but that this duty had not been breached. The Trust's system was accepted by the medical witnesses as appropriate. The delay was not felt to be unreasonable. The system had to accommodate that which was reasonably foreseeable rather than rare occurrences. Account had to be taken of the resources available in considering the standard of care.[64]

9.8.10 Of note, *Bull v Devon* (*see* Section 9.8.6) was not considered. This is one area of law that is likely to develop over time.[65]

---

62 *Jones v Manchester Corp* [1952] 2 All ER 125, CA.
63 [2006] EWHC 2314.
64 *See* also *Cowley v Cheshire & Merseyside Strategic Health Authority* [2007] EWHC 48.
65 *See*, for example, Beswick J. A first class service? Setting the standard of care for the contemporary NHS. *Med Law Rev.* 2007; 15(2): 245–52.

9.9 CONCLUSION

9.9.1 The duty of care is a core concept. It is the legal relationship between legal personae. The key is to recognise the existence of such legal connections and to understand what obligation is imposed by virtue of such relationships. It is important to realise that the obligation imposed may vary depending upon the nature of the legal connection.

10 Negligence: breach of the duty of care

10.1 GENERAL PRINCIPLES

10.1.1 In the previous sections we have seen that the existence of a doctor–patient relationship (medical professional–patient relationship) is sufficient to create **a duty of care**. We have considered the situations when a duty of care might arise. As we have seen, not all relationships amount to a doctor–patient relationship.

10.1.2 Knowing that you owe a duty of care to someone does not tell you what you have to do to discharge that duty. A duty of care contains certain obligations. This is the idea of the **content of a duty of care**, which tells you what should be done or not be done to discharge that duty of care.

10.1.3 To discover what should be done we need a yardstick by which to measure the content of the duty of care, some standard by which we can judge what should have been done. This yardstick is called the **standard of care**. The more stringent the standard, the harder it is to meet.

10.1.4 In negligence, a claim can only really arise when the duty is not satisfactorily discharged.[1] This is the idea of the **breach of the duty of care**. To determine whether a breach of the duty of care has occurred, the Court determines what actually happened, i.e. the facts of the case, by taking evidence. It then compares what actually happened with the standard of care which is required by the law. If what actually happened falls below what should have happened, then the Court can conclude that a breach of the duty of care has occurred. Note how the standard of care is a question of law.

10.1.5 The advent of an adverse outcome alone does not establish the existence of breach of the duty of care. Risks materialise in medical practice even when the utmost skill and attention is deployed. The reason for the principle of the breach of the duty of care is to distinguish

---

1 This could be either when what should be done is not done, or when what should not be done is done.

those situations where an adverse outcome is simply the chance materialisation of an existing risk from those situations where there the adverse outcome results because due skill and attention was not deployed.

Whitehouse v Jordan [1980] 1 All ER 650, HL

P's mother was in the late stages of labour. She was attended by D. D undertook a trial of forceps prior to delivering P by caesarean section. P suffered significant brain damage.

P sued by her mother as best friend claiming that the trial of forceps was negligently undertaken.

Held: D not liable.

10.1.6 The measure of the standard of care (i.e. what should have been done) is an objective question, and the answer should not depend upon the perspective from which the question is viewed. The standard of care is considered further in sections 10.3 and 10.4.

10.1.7 The idea of **reasonableness** is used to import this objectivity into the idea of the standard of care. This word 'reasonable' is not used in the everyday sense of being sensible. Here the term means ordinary, everyday, around the middle of the normal curve. It does not imply ideas of averaging, and it eschews the idea of extremes – but it does import an objective element.

10.2 THE REASONABLE PERSON STANDARD

10.2.1 The reasonable person standard is an elastic concept that adapts to the situation faced by the Court. It will consider all the circumstances of the case before deciding which reasonable person standard yardstick is applicable in that case. For example, in general cases the reasonable person has been described as a passenger on the Underground.[2] For cases involving persons possessing a particular skill, the reasonable person standard possesses the requisite skill to an ordinary level found in that profession.

---

2   *McFarlane v Tayside Health Board* [1999] 4 All ER 961.

10.2.2   The choice of which measure to use on this reasonable skilled person yardstick depends upon what the medical professional leads the patient to believe their professional skills are. This may be as a specialist, generalist, physician, nurse or indeed Chinese herbalist.

Shakoor v Situ [2000] 4 All ER 181

D was a qualified practitioner of traditional Chinese herbal medicine. D prescribed P a Chinese herbal remedy for a skin condition. Consequent to this P suffered an idiosyncratic drug reaction including acute liver-failure and later died, despite liver transplantation.

There had been papers in the western medical journals, including letters in the Lancet, describing liver failure in people treated with Chinese herbal remedies. D was unaware of these. D did, however, keep up to date with developments in Chinese herbal medicine.

Held: D did not breach the standard of care.

An ordinary skilled practitioner of traditional Chinese herbal medicine could not be expected to have read and taken notice of the letters in the Lancet.

The standard of the 'ordinary skilled [person] exercising and professing to have that special skill'[3] applies to all medical professionals.

10.2.3   To ensure that the level of care that a patient can expect does not depend upon the skills or experience of the particular doctor they see, the reasonable skilled person yardstick does not accommodate inexperience within posts. It sets itself by what the medical professional holds themselves out to be.[4] Therefore, within the NHS, an inexperienced doctor working in a post soon after promotion will not be judged by their particular attributes but by what might be expected from an ordinary skilled person who holds that particular post. This takes into account the differing or more advance skills required for particular or specialist posts.

---

3   *Bolam v Friern Hospital Management Committee* [1957] 2 All ER 118 per McNair J.
4   *Holton v General Medical Council* [2006] EWHC 2960, para. 71 per Stanley Burnton J.

Wilsher v Essex AHA [1986] 3 All ER 801, CA

A neonate born three months prematurely was attended by an inexperienced doctor (senior house officer (SHO)). Unfortunately the SHO misplaced the umbilical arterial catheter into a vein.[5] The SHO did check the position with a more senior doctor (the registrar), who also did not notice that the catheter had been misplaced. After about nine hours the catheter was replaced by the registrar, but was again erroneously placed into a vein.

As a result, the neonate received excess oxygen for 12–14 hours resulting in retrolental fibroplasia.

Held: The claim for breach of the duty of care was successful.

The test for the standard of care is not that of the average skilled SHO but of the average skilled SHO who fills the post in question.

The SHO did not breach the duty of care because he sought senior advice. However, the Registrar did breach his duty of care.

The case went to the House of Lords on a point pertaining to causation (*see* Section 11.2.4) where a retrial was ordered, but the case was settled before the retrial.

10.3 THE STANDARD OF CARE: THE *BOLAM* TEST

10.3.1 Having considered the standard by which a medical practitioner is judged, consider now the yardstick by which the actions of a medical practitioner can be judged. To arrive at this we begin with the famous *Bolam* standard:

> 'a doctor is not guilty of negligence if he acts in accordance with a practice accepted as proper by a responsible body of medical men skilled in that particular art . . .'[3]

Bolam v Friern Hospital Management Committee [1957] 2 All ER 118

D administered electroconvulsive therapy to P without administering muscle relaxant. Only the lower jaw was physically restrained. Patient suffered a fractured hip.

---

5   It seems that the tip of this catheter lodged in the left atrium having traversed the patent foramen ovale.

The patient sued the Hospital as vicariously liable (*see* para. 9.8.4) for the actions of D.

Jury: Returned a verdict in favour of D.

10.3.2 On this approach, if there were two legitimate schools of medical thought then provided the doctor acted within one school they would not be in breach of their duty of care.[6]

Maynard v West Midlands Regional HA [1985] 1 All ER 635, HL

P suffered mediastinal lymphadenopathy without pulmonary lesions. D felt that, although tuberculosis (TB) was most the most likely diagnosis, the differential diagnosis included Hodgkin's disease, carcinoma and sarcoidosis. D undertook biopsy to exclude Hodgkin's disease. To obtain this biopsy D undertook mediastinoscopy. Mediastinoscopy resulted in left recurrent laryngeal nerve paralysis.

P was, in fact, suffering from TB. P alleged that D should have diagnosed TB and not proceeded with the mediastinoscopy.

Medical evidence was available supporting D's approach. But there was another body of medical evidence suggesting that TB should have been treated without resorting to mediastinoscopy.

At first instance: D found negligent. The judge preferred the evidence of one body of medical experts.

Held: D not negligent.

The judge was not entitled to prefer one body of legitimate medical evidence over another.

10.4 THE NEW *BOLAM* TEST, *BOLAM* AFTER *BOLITHO*

10.4.1 The essence of the *Bolam* standard is that the yardstick by which medical professionals are judged is simply whether or not they follow the practice of a group of their peers. This approach has a profound weakness – there does not seem to be any clear objective element.

---

6   *Hunter v Hanley* 1955 SC 200.

10.4.2 The standard of care appears to rest purely upon medical judgement.[7] The mere opinions of doctors, however learned, are never sufficient alone to constitute factual truth. The learning of medical professionals may make it more likely that the truth will lie in the direction of their opinions, but this is not guaranteed.

10.4.3 The real question is: 'What *should* have happened here?'[8] The Court holds the final decision in relation to this question. Thus, it can conclude that a course of action acceptable to a reasonable body of medical opinion is not one that meets standard of care required to discharge the legal duty of care.

Hucks v Cole (1968) (1993) 4 Med LR 393, CA

P had the rash of puerperal fever (post-partum septicemia) secondary to *Streptococcus pyogenes* infection. D failed to treat P with the bacteriocidal antibiotic penicillin, instead choosing to use the bacteriostatic antibiotic tetracycline.

After a five day course P was discharged with evidence of persisting infection. She went on to suffer fulminating septicaemia.

A body of medical opinion supported D's action, although the Court found that it was not a matter of two schools of medical thought, rather another doctor's opinion that he, too, might have acted the same way as D had in the circumstances.

Held: D negligent for not treating with penicillin, given the evidence of persisting infection after the course of tetracycline.

10.4.4 The Court is seeking to arrive at the truth of the matter. It accepts its limitations in that it cannot bring to bear on cases involving medical issues the years of medical training, skill and experience that expert medical practitioners have at their disposal. However, there is a line between relying upon medical knowledge supported by its evidence base (such as it is) and relying upon mere unsupported medical

---

7 *Sidaway v Board of Governors of the Bethlem Royal Hospital* [1985] 1 All ER 643, 644 per Scarmen Ld.

8 Hurwicz B. Clinical guidelines: legal and political considerations of clinical practice guidelines. *BMJ*. 1999; **318**: 661.

opinion.[9] For these reasons, *inter alia*, the *Bolam* standard was restated in *Bolitho v City & Hackney HA*.[10]

Bolitho v City & Hackney HA [1997] UKHL 46, HL

A 2-year-old child suffering from croup had two cyanotic episodes. D failed to attend. P suffered an episode of respiratory failure and cardiac arrest soon after the second episode. P was resuscitated but had suffered severe brain damage and subsequently died.

If intubated before the third episode the cardiac arrest would not have occurred.

D said that if she had attended she would have decided not to intubate.

A reasonable body of medical opinion supported D's view that a decision not to intubate accorded with acceptable medical practice, although there was a body of medical opinion taking the other view.

Held: The failure to attend P was negligent (i.e. a breach of the duty of care). In light of the medical evidence, a decision not to intubate P would not have been negligent.

Given the latter finding, it was not possible to establish that the negligent failure to attend caused the cardiac arrest. This would have occurred in any case had P attended and then decided not to intubate.

P's claim failed on causation (*see* Section 11.4).

10.4.5 Caught in the midst of conflicting medical opinions, the weakness of the pure *Bolam* standard was addressed first to the Court of Appeal[11] and then in the House of Lords in *Bolitho*. Their conclusion was that the exponents of a body of medical opinion must be able to demonstrate that their opinion had a logical basis. They approved the decision in *Hucks v Cole* (*see* Section 10.4.3).

10.4.6 The test for the standard of medical care is now a modification of the pure *Bolam* standard and can be stated as:

> A doctor is not guilty of negligence if he acts in accordance with a practice accepted as proper by a **reasonable, responsible** and **respectable body** of medical men skilled in that particular art.

---

9   Woolf H. Are the courts excessively deferential to the medical profession? *Med Law Rev.* 2001; 9(1): 1–16.
10   [1997] UKHL 46.
11   Bolitho v City & Hackney HA (1993) 13 BMLR 111, CA.

10.4.7   Note how the words 'reasonable' and 'responsible' have been introduced into the standard, importing an objective element (*see* Section 10.1.7) into the *Bolam* test thereby detaching it from resting purely upon received medical opinion. In light of this, a judge can choose not to accept a body of medical opinion evidence that is not coherent when subject to logical analysis. Such a situation would only arise on rare occasions. This does not make the decision in *Maynard v West Midlands Regional HA* (*see* Section 10.3.2) incorrect. It does, however, leave the Court with the option to explore the cogency of the medical evidence presented, with the option of not accepting it if that evidence lacks a logical basis.

10.4.8   This principle can extend to cover a hospital's duty of care. Thus, if a hospital policy has a logical basis and accords with the modified *Bolam* standard (*see* Section 10.4.6), i.e. falling within a range of reasonable policies, very seldom will a situation arise when the hospital will be found to breach the duty of care.[12]

10.5   CONCLUSION

10.5.1   Where the obligation imposed by a duty of care has not been met that duty is said to have been breached. Whether a breach has occurred or not requires careful factual and legal analysis. In many medical cases the question turns upon the Court's view of the medical evidence and the requisite standard of care in the circumstances in question.

---

12   *Cowley v Cheshire & Merseyside Strategic Health Authority* [2007] EWHC 48.

11 Causation

11.1 INTRODUCTION

11.1.1 We have now established that negligence arises where a legal obligation to act or not act (a duty of care) is breached. A claim in negligence is to recover damages to compensate the victim for some harm that has been suffered, but the party owing the duty of care does not insure the claimant for all harm suffered. It is unjust to require someone to compensate another for harm they have not caused.[1] Therefore, it is necessary to identify some damage that has been suffered and then demonstrate that that damage is causally related to the breach of duty that has occurred.

11.1.2 The basic principle can be stated as follows:

> If causation is established then P can recover in full for the harm. If the connection between the breach and the harm is not established, then P can recover nothing for the harm.

The apparent harshness of this test has been examined in the case law but, after much consideration, the balance of the argument fell in favour of a 'bright line' rule. This promotes certainty and clarity, on occasion at the expense of justice, but the rule has been softened in certain areas (*see* Sections 6.5, 11.5 and 11.6) to accommodate its potential for injustice.

11.1.3 The burden is upon the person seeking damages to establish that the breach of the duty of care complained about is causally related to the damage complained about.[2] They must establish on a balance of probabilities (i.e. more than 50% likely) that the breach of the duty of care caused the damage complained about.

---

1   *Fairchild v Glenhaven Funeral Services Ltd* [2002] UKHL 22 at para. 33 per Bingham Ld.
2   *Wilsher v Essex AHA* [1988] 1 All ER 871, HL.

Loveday v Renton (1990) 1 Med LR 117, CA

This was a class action. P were about 200 claimants who had suffered brain damage after receiving pertussis vaccine. On the basis of medical case reports and other medical evidence describing a temporal relationship between the vaccination and brain damage, P alleged that the brain damage flowed from receiving the pertussis vaccine.

Held: P did not recover.

The scientific evidence did not establish on a balance of probabilities a causal link between brain damage and the pertussis vaccine in young children. The clinical proof had to equate to the balance of probabilities standard.

11.2 THE 'BUT–FOR' TEST

11.2.1   The core principle used to establishing a causal link is the **but–for** test:[3]

    (i) If the damage would have resulted with the breach of the duty of care, and

    (ii) the damage would not have resulted in the absence of the breach of the duty of care,

  then

    (iii) the breach of the duty of caused the damage.

11.2.2   Clearly this could be incorrect if the breach of duty was subject to a confounding variable, but common sense is added when interpreting this test.

11.2.3   Using this definition, if the outcome would be the same whether there was a breach of the duty of care or not, then the breach did not cause the harm complained about. This is demonstrated by the facts of *Barnett v Chelsea & Kensington Hospital Management Committee* (*see* Section 9.2.1). Here the nightwatchman attended the accident and emergency department but was not seen by a doctor. The failure to attend the patient was a breach of the duty of care. However, it was found that even if the watchman had been seen by the doctor the

---

3   Also known as *causa sine qua non*.

watchman would still have died of arsenic poisoning. The breach did not cause the death of the watchman.

11.2.4   If there is more than one way by which the harm could have arisen and it is not possible to establish on a balance of probabilities that the harm complained about resulted from the breach of duty then causation is not established and the case fails.

Wilsher v Essex AHA [1988] 1 All ER 871, HL

P was a neonate requiring respiratory support. Blood gas monitoring was conducted via an umbilical arterial catheter. Unfortunately, this was misplaced into an umbilical vein resulting in neonatal hyperoxia. P suffered retrolental fibroplasia ('RLF').

Medical evidence supported the conclusion that a sufficiently high p_aO_2 for a sufficiently long period can affect the retinal vessels. These changes may regress or progress to RLF. There remained two matters of controversy between the medical witnesses: the actual level of hyperoxia P was exposed to (because the only available blood gas results for that period were venous samples), and the contribution to the retrolental fibroplasia made by the other conditions suffered by P (apnoea, hypercarbia, intraventricular haemorrhage and patent ductus arteriosus).

The trial at first instance (Peter Pain J) had been held on the assumption that the burden of proving that the breach had not caused the RLF fell on D rather than P.

Held: P did not recover because causation had not been established. The burden of proving causation falls on P. Insufficient evidence was adduced by P to prove on a balance of probabilities that causation had been established. But given that the wrong assumption was made in relation to the burden of proof at first instance, P's claim could not be dismissed. A retrial was ordered (*see*, also, Section 10.2.3).

11.3   LOSS OF CHANCE IS NOT RECOVERABLE

11.3.1   One key question is what is the harm? Losing the chance of getting something is not the same as losing that thing. Because negligence is about compensating for harm that has occurred, it is the loss of the thing that is compensated for not the loss of the chance of the thing.

The gist of negligence is damage.[4] In relation to medical claims this is a crucial point to grasp.

Hotson v East Berkshire AHA [1987] 2 All ER 909, HL

P fell out of a tree and suffered a fracture of the left femoral epiphysis. D failed to diagnose the injury. The injury was diagnosed and treated later. P suffered avascular necrosis of the hip.

The medical evidence was that if P had been diagnosed initially there was a 75% chance that he would still have suffered avascular necrosis of the hip but, with prompt treatment, there was a 25% chance of a full recovery. With the delay he had a 100% chance of avascular necrosis of the hip.

Held CA: P had lost a 25% chance of full recovery so awarded P 25% of his calculated damages.

Held HL (unanimously): P could not recover at all.

11.3.2   To make sense of *Hotson* look at **Figure 1** (page 136). Here the breach was the delay in diagnosis and the harm complained about was the avascular necrosis of the hip. In the presence of the delay there was a 100% chance of avascular necrosis of the hip. But in the absence of the breach there was still a 75% chance that avascular necrosis would result.

11.3.3   The point is that, on a balance of probabilities, even if the breach had not occurred there was a 75% that the avascular necrosis would still have occurred. This conclusion is coupled with a second rule that if causation is established P recovers for all his damage, whilst if causation is not established P recovers nothing. The basis of this second rule is that it promotes certainty and prevents P only being partially compensated for the spurious reason that the causal connection cannot be established with certainty. The latter point is particularly important in medical cases, where it is rare to establish causation with absolute certainty.

11.3.4   The result is a feeling of injustice flowing from sound reasoning. This feeling of injustice arises because there is another view of this type of situation: that the damage is not the avascular necrosis of the hip but is, in fact, the 25% lost chance of a complete recovery. If the damage

---

4   Stapleton J. The gist of negligence. *LQR.* 1998; **104:** 389, 391–2.

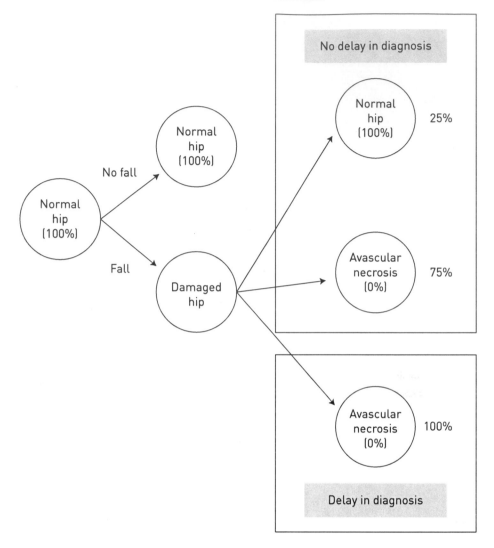

Figure 1 No recovery for loss of chance – *Hotson v East Berkshire AHA*. The numbers on the circles represent the fitness of the hip – 100% is a fully fit hip. Notice how the delay in diagnosis converted a 25% chance of complete recovery into a 0% chance of complete recovery. The but–for rule of causation requires on a balance of probabilities that, but–for the breach, the harm would not have arisen. Here in the absence of the delay there is 75% chance P would have suffered avascular necrosis of the hip in any case therefore causation was not established.

is this lost chance, then it is easier to establish that it is causally related to the breach.[5] This view was rejected unanimously by the House of Lords for the physical injury suffered in *Hotson*. But the debate was revisited in the recent case of *Gregg v Scott*.[6] In this case, a bare majority (3:2) of the House of Lords also rejected this view.

Gregg v Scott [2005] UKHL 2

Hoffmann Ld, Phillips Ld, Baroness Hale, Nicholls Ld (Dissent),Hope Ld (Dissent)

P was suffering from non-Hodgkin's lymphoma[7] (NHL), a form of haematological malignancy. In essence, D delayed the diagnosis of P's NHL by nine months. The likelihood of 10-year disease-free survival was found to have been reduced from 42% to 25% by the delay. Of note, at the time of the trial, approximately nine years after the breach of care, P was alive and in remission.

P claimed only for the lifespan lost as a result of the breach.[8] P did not claim for physical damage suffered as a result of the breach.

Held: P could not recover for loss of chance.

Majority: *Hoffmann Ld, Phillips Ld* and *Baroness Hale* agreed that the weight of authority should not be overturned. *Baroness Hale:* Allowing loss of chance would be likely to be unjust to those in the majority of cases – they would only partially recover for want of certain causation. It would also reduce the certainty prized by the legal process. *Phillips Ld:* Proof of causation is about providing evidence of a causal link. The evidence is not the link itself. Once proven to the requisite standard, the link is taken to exist and full recovery is permitted. Given that P was alive after nine years despite the delay in treatment, it was likely he was in the survivors group from the very beginning.

Dissenting: *Nicholls Ld:* The rule precluding recovery for loss of chance was unjust and should be abandoned.

Hope Ld: P could recover for the physical damage flowing from the breach.

---

5   This view has been accepted in relation to economic loss: *Chaplin v Hicks* [1911] 2 KB 786; *Kitchen v Royal Air Force Association* [1958] 1 WLR 563; *Spring v Guardian Assurance PLC* [1994] 3 All ER 129, 153; *Allied Maples Group Ltd v Simmons & Simmons* [1995] 1 WLR 1602.

6   [2005] UKHL 2.

7   Anaplastic Lymphoma Kinase (ALK) Negative.

8   'Lost years' – *Pickett v British Rail Engineering* [1980] AC 136.

11.3.5   The concept of causation appears to be a deterministic one. Whatever knowledge we had about P, from the beginning P was destined to survive or not-survive. The object of the evidence is to persuade the Court, on a balance of probabilities, that the breach caused or would cause P to move from the survivor to the non-survivor group. The idea that causation operates partially, in a degree determined by the evidence available, was rejected. The net result is that full recovery is permitted where it can be demonstrated, on a balance of probabilities, that the breach caused the harm complained about.

It is an important observation that a predictive statistical model based on previous cases and the actual damage suffered by P are different things. It is an error to confuse probabilities based on observations in other cases for a certain prediction about cause and effect in a particular case.[9]

11.4   CAUSATION IN CASES OF BREACH OF DUTY BY OMISSION

11.4.1   Breach of duty can be by commission, i.e. doing something you should not do, or by omission, i.e. not doing something you should have done because there was a duty to act. Establishing a causal connection between a breach and the harm complained about in cases of omission raises particular issues.

11.4.2   When applying the but–for test, notice how there is a comparison of two limbs (*see* **Figure 2**, p. 139):

(i) What did happen?

and

(ii) What would have happened if the negligence had not occurred?

11.4.3   Consider the second limb. What if there is a choice to be made by D in this second hypothetical limb? Such a situation may arise where the breach was an omission.

11.4.4   In *Bolitho* (*see* Section 10.4.4) the doctor should have attended the child but did not. We know that the child suffered respiratory arrest when they were not attended (*see* **Figure 2**, p. 139). In considering what would have happened if the child had been attended, we ask a

---

9   *Meadow v General Medical Council* [2006] EWHC 146 (Admin). *See*, also, Devaney S. The loneliness of the expert witness. *General Medical Council v Meadow. Med Law Rev.* 2007; **15**(1): 116–25.

second question of the respondent, D: 'If you had attended, then what would you have done?'

11.4.5   The choice is between whether to intubate or not to intubate. Intubation would have prevented the third respiratory arrest, but this is with the benefit of hindsight. In this case, D said that if they had attended the child they would have chosen not to intubate. The medical evidence supported this action, i.e. this decision would not have constituted a breach of the duty of care and there was no negligence in making this choice. Thus, the only breach was the failure to attend and this failure to attend was not causally related to the harm.

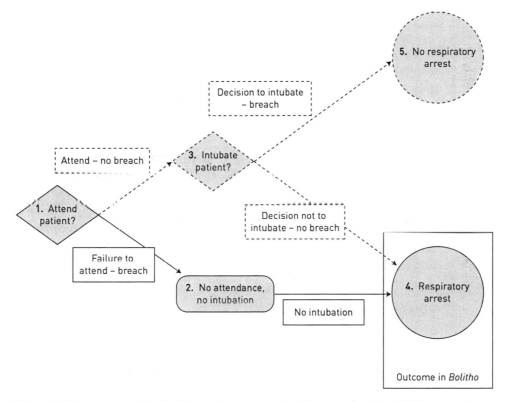

Figure 2 The causal chain in *Bolitho* (*see* Sections 11.3 *et seq.*) with solid lines marking actual events and dotted lines marking hypothetical connections. Notice how only attending the child *plus* a decision to intubate (1→3→5) could have prevented the respiratory arrest. Thus the failure to attend alone was not sufficient to cause the respiratory arrest. Thus, the hypothetical decision not to intubate (3→4) is a critical step in determining whether the failure to attend was or was not causally related to the respiratory arrest.

11.4.6   If it would have been negligent not to intubate then P could not argue that they would have chosen not to intubate. In this alternative scenario the failure to attend would be casually related to the harm. From this we can see that in cases of omission it is possible to establish causation in two ways, i.e. by demonstrating either that:

(i) in the event D would have done something (e.g. intubation) that would have avoided the harm, or

(ii) it would have been negligent for D not to do the thing that avoided the harm.[10]

This is because if D had chosen not to do the thing that avoided the harm (e.g. chosen not to intubate as in *Bolitho*) then the medical professional can only avoid negligence if this choice would have been in accordance with their duty of care.

11.4.7 The result in (i) is open to two criticisms. Firstly that D will be answering a hypothetical question, knowing that their choice might affect the outcome of the case. Secondly that it falls to P to prove what D would have done had they attended, whereas D is much better placed to answer this question.

11.4.8 If P is unable to leap the hurdle set by (i) then P must fall back on to option (ii). This leaves P in a position where they must prove that D's failure to intubate lacked a logical basis. If D has the body of medical opinion in support of their position (i.e. supporting the decision not to intubate) then P is left to demonstrate that this body of medical opinion lacks a logical basis. This is a heavy burden of proof to discharge.[11]

11.4.9 Despite this evidentiary difficulty, the logic operates in other cases of breach by omission.

Joyce v Merton, Sutton and Wandsworth HA (1996) 7 Med LR 1,CA[12]

D performed cardiac catheterisation using the right brachial artery for access to the circulation. After the procedure the brachial artery was closed using sutures. D inadvertently sutured the anterior wall of the brachial artery to the intima of the posterior wall. No problem was noted at that time. P was discharged the following day.

12 days later P was seen in OPD and right brachial artery occlusion was noted. P was, therefore, referred for a vascular surgical opinion. Despite

---

10   *Joyce v Merton, Sutton and Wandsworth HA* (1996) 7 Med LR 1 per Hobhouse LJ.
11   *Zarb v Odetoyinbo* [2006] EWHC 2880.
12   *See* Grubb A. Medical negligence: breach of duty and causation. *Med Law Rev.* 1996; 4: 86.

vascular reconstruction, P's arm did not improve. A subsequent arch aortogram dislodged thrombus resulting in an upper brainstem stroke and subsequent locked-in syndrome.

It was accepted that re-exploration of the arm within 48 hours would have prevented the need for further surgery and the arch aortogram.

D admitted the suturing error. Medical evidence was that this could have occurred without negligent performance of the technique. The evidence of the vascular surgeons was that they would not have operated within 48 hours if they had seen P within that window of time.

Held: P could not recover.

D was not negligent in the suturing or in discharging P because it was unlikely on the medical evidence that there would have been signs that would have justified further action prior to discharge.

D was negligent in that the instructions given to P prior to discharge, in relation to returning if there were problems, were not adequate. However, it was not possible to create a causal link between this breach and the subsequent damage on the evidence.

11.4.10   In other situations the material hypothetical choice is not that of the medical profession omitting to act but, in fact, the choice that would have been made by someone else. In *Zarb v Odetoyinbo*[13] a GP did not promptly refer a patient with back pain for urgent neurosurgical assessment. The patient suffered *cauda equina* syndrome despite surgical decompression (L4 laminectomy). The neurosurgeon who might have received an urgent referral from the GP was not identified, so the first part of the test could not be met (*see* para. 11.4.6). The second part of the test was not met either because the medical evidence was held not to demonstrate that neurosurgery would have been mandated had the GP promptly referred. Given the fact that the duty of the neurosurgeon, in accordance with the modified *Bolam* standard, did not mandate immediate surgery, then the duty of the GP could not extend to require immediate referral and so the GP was not in breach of duty.

---

13   [2006] EWHC 2880.

11.5 INNOCENT AND GUILTY CAUSES

11.5.1 In some cases the damage complained about can be caused by multiple mechanisms. If some of these mechanisms are guilty mechanisms and others are innocent mechanisms then it can become difficult to formally satisfy the but–for test (*see* Section 11.2). In some situations the Court has accepted as a causal connection a test that is less stringent than the but–for test, particularly for industrial injury cases (*see* Section 11.6.7).

11.5.2 Broadly speaking, it may be sufficient to establish causation where a guilty cause makes either:

(i) a material contribution to the magnitude of the harm, or

(ii) a material contribution to the risk of the harm.

11.5.3 The but–for test remains logically the strongest evidence of causation and akin to the logic of Koch's postulates.[14] It establishes *factual* causation. These other means to establish causation are accepted as sufficient to establish *legal* causation. The inherent evidential gap between the but–for test and the other means to establish causation was accepted, possibly on pragmatic grounds[15] but also on the balance of injustice.

11.5.4 **Material contribution to the harm:** Where there is more than one potential cause for the harm complained about and the contribution of each cause to that harm cannot be quantified because of the current state of medical science it is not necessary to establish that the guilty cause was wholly responsible for the harm complained about.[16]

11.5.5 It is sufficient to show, on a balance of probabilities that the guilty cause materially contributed to the harm complained about.

---

14 To identify pathogenic organisms: (1) The organism must be isolated from a diseased animal and grown in a pure culture. (2) The cultured organism should cause disease when introduced into a healthy animal. And (3) the organism must be re-isolated from the experimentally infected animal.

15 *McGhee v National Coal Board* [1972] 3 All ER 1008, 1010 per Reid Ld; *Alphacell Ltd v Woodward* [1972] 2 All ER 475, 489 per Salmon Ld.

16 *McGhee v National Coal Board* [1972] 3 All ER 1008, 1009 per Reid Ld.

Bonnington Castings Ltd v Wardlaw [1956] 1 All ER 615,[17] HL

P worked for D for 8 years in a foundry making steel castings. P operated a pneumatic hammer. Over the period of his employment P was exposed to silica dust from two sources:

(i) swing grinders whose dust-extraction facility was not fully operational in breach of duty[18] (the guilty source), and

(ii) pneumatic hammers against the dust from which there was no known protection at the time (the innocent source).

There was no evidence to show the proportions in which the dust emanated from the innocent and the guilty source. As a result of the exposure to the silica dust P developed a pneumoconiosis.

Held: D could recover.

A material contribution[19] by guilty cause was sufficient to discharge burden of proving causation.

11.5.6   The question here is magnitude of the contribution to the harm made by the guilty cause, i.e. how much worse did the harm become? If it was materially worse then the link is established. Thus the guilty silica in P's lungs in the *Bonnington Castings* case was present in addition to the innocent dust that P had inhaled. This additional guilty silica materially contributed to the harm of damaging P's lungs.

11.5.7   **Material contribution to the risk of harm:** There are situations where medical uncertainty is such that it is impossible to say for certain that a particular guilty cause materially contributed to the harm complained about. In such cases if the harm suffered by P falls squarely within the risk created by D's breach[20] and it is possible to say that the guilty cause materially increased the risk of that harm developing then causation may be established.

---

17   *See,* also, *Nicholson v Atlas Steel Foundry and Engineering Co Ltd* [1957] 1 All ER 776. Similar outcome, similar facts.

18   In fact, this was a statutory duty.

19   'Material' seems to mean only more than *de minimis. Bonnington Castings Ltd v Wardlaw* [1956] 1 All ER 615, 618 per Reid Ld.

20   *McGhee v National Coal Board* [1972] 3 All ER 1008, 1012 per Wilberforce Ld.

McGhee v National Coal Board [1972] 3 All ER 1008, HL

For many years P was a labourer at a brickworks where he was exposed to brick dust. His employer (D) failed to provide P with showering facilities to wash off the brick dust. This failure to provide showers was held to be a breach of the duty of care D owed P. As a result of this breach of duty P had to cycle home covered in brick dust before he could remove the brick dust from his skin.

The brick dust adhered to his skin causing dermatitis. It was agreed that the dermatitis was caused by the brick dust. The medical causal relationship between the brick dust and the dermatitis was not fully understood. But it was established that the added duration of exposure to the brick dust would be likely to increase to risk of developing dermatitis.

The medical evidence was that:

It could not be established that if showers had been provided it was more probable than not that the dermatitis would have been avoided.

The provision of showers would have materially reduced the risk of developing dermatitis.

Held: P could recover.

11.5.8   Here the the guilty cause has made the harm more likely without making the harm better or worse. It was the brick dust that caused the dermatitis. But the guilty brick dust was exactly the same brick dust that was innocent brick dust before the point in time that P should have been able to take his shower. The longer P was exposed to the brick dust the more likely he was to suffer dermatitis. We cannot say that the dermatitis was worse because the brick dust was present on the skin longer, only that P was more likely to get dermatitis because the brick dust was on his skin longer.

11.5.9   In *McGhee* the Court of Appeal applied the but–for test and refused to allow P to recover damages. The House of Lords overturned this decision extending the concept of causation in law for negligence cases beyond the but–for principle.[21] Interestingly this was the rule applied by the Court of Appeal in *Wilsher* (*see* Section 11.2.4) but rejected in favour of the but–for test by the House of Lords.

---

21   *Fairchild v Glenhaven Funeral Services Ltd* [2002] UKHL 22.

11.6 MULTIPLE GUILTY CAUSES AND MULTIPLE RESPONDENTS (D1, D2, D3 ETC.)

11.6.1 Where there are multiple respondents each of whom has materially contributed[22] to a single, indivisible injury then the claimant (P) can recover the whole of his damages from any one of them. As between the respondents, they can sue one other for a contribution to the damages paid to P. In such cases all the respondents can be joined in a single legal action.[23] Each respondent is held liable in proportion to the amount of risk they created.[22]

11.6.2 In general if P cannot establish which respondent's breach was causally related to the damage complained about then P's case fails. This can create injustice in some circumstances. Particularly where medical science is not yet in a position to identify which breach caused the harm. In such cases the Court can leap the evidential gap in the interests of justice permitting P to recover even without formally establishing causation.

Fairchild v Glenhaven Funeral Services Ltd [2002] UKHL 22, HL

P[24] was employed by two employers (D1 and D2). P was employed for different periods with each employer. Each employer was in breach of their duty to prevent P from inhaling asbestos dust. During the time with each employer P had inhaled excessive asbestos dust. P had no other exposure to asbestos. P developed mesothelioma, became terminally ill and subsequently died.

It was found that the mesothelioma was caused by the asbestos exposure. The risk of mesothelioma increased with an increased amount of asbestos inhaled. The medical evidence was that the possibility that any single fibre may have caused the condition was as likely as the possibility that many fibres together had caused the condition.

Actions were brought on behalf of P by the estates of P. P could not prove on a balance of probabilities whether the asbestos causing the mesothelioma had been inhaled at one or other of the employers.

---

22 *Barker v Corus (UK) Ltd* [2006] UKHL 20; [2006] 3 All ER 785, HL.
23 *See* Rogers WVH. *Winfield & Jolowicz on Tort.* 17th ed. London: Sweet & Maxwell; 2006. p.919 *et seq.*
24 In fact, there were three appeals. In two cases the plaintiff had already died; in the third, the plaintiff was alive but suffering from mesothelioma.

Court of Appeal:[25] P could not recover because the 'but–for' test had not been satisfied.

Held HL: P could recover.

11.6.3   In *Fairchild*[26] the Court accepted that neither could the but–for test be satisfied nor could it be demonstrated that the breach materially contributed to the harm. Despite this the Court resiled at the idea that both D1 and D2 could avoid liability by arguing that they were both in breach of their duty of care.

11.6.4   If D1 and D2 had been a single employer P would have been able to recover. However given the state of medical knowledge it was impossible to prove whether it was asbestos from D1's breach, D2's breach or both breaches that had caused P's mesothelioma. Justice demanded that P should be able to recover.

11.6.5   The difficulty was that whilst it was just for P to recover it was unjust for an employer to pay damages for something that they had not caused. The Court therefore considered the balance of injustice. In this case the Court favoured the lesser injustice of making the employers liable for the breach they had committed without strict proof of causation over the greater injustice of leaving P, who had suffered mesothelioma as a result of their asbestos exposure, without a remedy.

11.6.6   However the nature of case law is that exceptions to the general rules of causation can expand and impose unforeseen liabilities as subsequent cases are decided. Therefore the Court laid down restrictions that might operate to limit this exception and its inherent injustice. P can recover where P can demonstrate that:

(i)   a duty of care exists and is owed by each of the respondents to P

(ii)   breach of this duty creates a risk to P

(iii)   that duty has been breached by each of the respondents

(iv)   the harm that resulted was within the area of risk created by the breach of duty of each of the respondents and that other causes

---

25   [2001] EWCA Civ 1881.
26   Followed in *Barker v Saint-Gobain Pipelines plc* [2005] 3 All ER 661, CA on similar facts.

are not operating (unlike the situation in *Wilsher* (*see* Section 11.2.4)), and

(v) medical science cannot identify which respondent's breach in fact caused the harm.

11.6.7 The House of Lords approved its decision in *Wilsher* in this case. The apparent restriction of the rule to cases involving industrial injury is not fully explicable except on policy grounds.[27]

11.6.8 There is another exception to the rule that causation must be proved in order to recover damages in negligence but this will be considered in the section on negligent misstatement which best falls to be considered under the rules surrounding consent[28] (*see* Section 6.4).

11.7 CONCLUSION

11.7.1 Like medical causation the basic concept of legal causation is a factual causal connection. There are differences however. The medical model of causation is based on propensity whilst the legal model is deterministic. This is mainly because medical professionals tend to view probabilities antecedent to the event whilst lawyers generally view probabilities after the event. Finally the legal model is, on occasion, distorted from being purely factual by the legal (and indeed moral) principle of justice.

---

27   *Fairchild v Glenhaven Funeral Services Ltd* [2002] UKHL 22, para. 69 per Hoffman Ld.
28   *Chester v Afshar* [2004] UKHL 41.

12 Legal status of the fetus

12.12.1 In case law a fetus only acquires a full legal status and protection if it is born alive.[1,2] Because it lacks legal status *in utero* it cannot be the victim of a crime of violence.[3] However, once it is born alive it acquires full legal status and the harm it suffers is recognised by law.[4]

12.12.2 The principle dates from the mid-17th century:[5]

> 'If a woman be quick with childe, and by a potion or otherwise killeth it in her wombe, or if a man beat her, whereby the childe dyeth in her body, and she is delivered of a deade childe, this is [...] no murder; but if the childe be born alive and dyeth of the potion, battery or other cause, this is murder; for in law it is accounted a reasonable creature [...] when it is born alive.'

12.12.3 An injury suffered whilst *in utero* can give rise to legal action where there is harm suffered after the delivery of the living child that is causally connect to the pre-delivery insult causing that harm.[3,6]

A-G's Reference (No.3 of 1994) **[1997] 3 All ER 936, HL**

V1 was approximately 24 weeks pregnant with her child V2. D, the natural father, stabbed V1 in the face, back and abdomen, intending only to harm V1. Both V1 and V2 survived the attack but two weeks later V1 delivered V2. V2 was born alive but prematurely. V2's chances of survival as a result of her prematurity were estimated at 50%.

After birth it became clear that one of the knife cuts had injured V2 such that she required surgical repair. V2 survived 121 days. Her cause of death was broncho-pulmonary dysplasia. The knife injury was not proved to have made any contribution to V2's subsequent death.

D was sentenced to four years imprisonment for wounding V1 with intention to cause grievous bodily harm.

---

1   [1680] 3 Coke, Institutes 50.
2   *Burton v Islington Health Authority* [1992] 3 All ER 833.
3   *A-G's Reference (No.3 of 1994)* [1997] 3 All ER 936.
4   *C v S* [1987] 1 All ER 1230; *Paton v Trustees of BPAS* [1978] 2 All ER 987.
5   [1680] 3 Coke, Institutes 50.
6   *R v Senior* (1832) 168 ER 1298; *Cherry v Borsman* (1991) 75 DLR (4th) 668.

After the death of V2, D was charged with the murder of V2 on the basis that the attack on V1 had caused the premature delivery. There was medical evidence causally linking the knife injuries and the premature delivery.

At trial D was acquitted of this charge.

The Attorney General referred the case for further opinion in relation to whether or not an injury to a fetus *in utero* could give rise to the crime of murder or manslaughter.

Held: Not murder because D lacked sufficient intention.[7]

But where there was an unlawful act that caused death, albeit unintentionally, this could constitute the crime of unlawful act manslaughter.[8] Therefore, in this case, if the causal connection between D's unlawful act and the death of V2 could be proved then it would be open to a jury to convict D of unlawful act manslaughter. It could not have been either murder or manslaughter if V2 had not been born alive.

12.12.4 In this case Ld Mustill took the view that the fetus is not a part of the mother: it is a distinct entity that exists in a symbiotic relationship with the mother.

12.12.5 Whilst the case law does not grant the fetus *in utero* the status of a legal entity, there are statutory provisions that do provide protection to the fetus. Except in certain circumstances, it is a criminal offence to procure or perform an abortion. Section 58 of the *Offences Against the Person Act 1861* makes it unlawful for anyone, including the pregnant woman, to procure a miscarriage.[9]

12.12.6 It has been concluded that miscarriage can only occur *after* the implantation of the fertilised ovum into the endometrium of the uterus. This has the important consequence of making most post-coital forms of

---

7 The doctrine of transferred malice was insufficient here. The doctrine needed to transfer D's intention to cause harm to V1 into an intention to cause harm to the fetus, V2 (which lacked legal existence at the time of the attack and so could not be the victim of the crime of murder) and thence to an intention to cause harm to the yet-to-be-born child, V2. (*A-G's Reference (No.3 of 1994)* [1997] 3 All ER 936, 948 per Mustill Ld).

8 In other words, D did not intend to harm V2, but his act was unlawful and likely to cause harm to someone which is a sufficient nexus of facts to establish the crime of manslaughter. Another situation where causing death unintentionally can amount to manslaughter is manslaughter by gross negligence: *R v Adomako* (*see* Section 8.2.1).

9 Note this does not make unlawful the more fanciful, but now not inconceivable, possibility of terminating a pregnancy borne by a man.

contraception lawful, including the morning-after pill and intrauterine devices.[10,11]

12.12.7 Added to this provision is the crime of child destruction created by Section 1 of the *Infant Life (Preservation) Act 1929*. This makes it a criminal offence to intentionally cause the death of a child capable of being born alive before the child has an existence independent of its mother.

12.12.8 The effect of this is to grant additional protection to a fetus that has the potential to survive independently from its mother. The statute does also provide an exception: that it must be proved that the act causing the child's death was not done in good faith and solely to preserve the life of the mother.

12.12.9 The maximum punishment for both these offences is life imprisonment, placing them on a par with the crime of manslaughter.

12.12.10 By section 1(2) of the *Infant Life (Preservation) Act 1929* there is a presumption that the child is capable of being born alive from 28 weeks of gestation. Capable of being born alive means being capable of 'living by reason of its breathing through its own lungs alone, without deriving any of its living or power of living by or through any connection with its mother'.[12]

12.12.11 By contrast, a 'stillborn' child is 'a child which has issued forth from its mother after the twenty-fourth week of pregnancy and which did not at any time after being completely expelled from its mother breathe or show any signs of life'.[13]

12.12.12 Whilst making clear that the fetus does not possess an absolute right to life,[14] the European Court of Human Rights has stubbornly refused to express an opinion on whether the fetus is covered by the Article 2: right to life at all, or whether it is covered but has limited rights.[15,16] Nor has it expressed an opinion on whether the unborn child is a legal person for the purposes of the Article 2: right to life.[17] It leaves the time at which the right to life begins to operate to be determined by

---

10   *R v Dhingra* (unreported) – *see Smeaton v Secretary of State for Health* [2002] EWHC 610.
11   *Smeaton v Secretary of State for Health* [2002] EWHC 610 (Admin).
12   *Rance v Mid-Downs HA* [1991] 1 All ER 801; *see*, also, *C v S* [1987] 1 All ER 1230.
13   s 41 *Births and Deaths Registration Act 1953*, as amended.
14   *X v United Kingdom* (1981) 3 EHRR 244, para. 12.
15   *Vö v France* [2004] ECHR 326.
16   O'Donovan K. Taking a neutral stance on the legal protection of the fetus. *Vö v France*. *Med Law Rev.* 2006; 14(1): 115–23.
17   *Vö v France* [2004] ECHR 326, para. 85.

national legal rules.[18,19] This is because it recognises the area of law as contentious and grants the signatory Nation States a wide margin of appreciation in relation[20] to determining when life begins. Therefore, if it exists, the fetal right to life is not contravened by the present English legal structure including the rules permitting abortion.[21]

12.12.13 The maternal right to respect for their private life (Article 8) encompasses the right to physical integrity (*see* Section 5.5.5).[22] This right does not form a basis to extend the rights of pregnant mothers to have access to abortions because the pregnancy entwines the mother's private life with that of the fetus.[23] However, where the law permits therapeutic abortion in circumstances where there is a threat to the mother's health, then the Article 8 right does require procedures that actually permit access to the possibility of therapeutic abortion even when a single specialist and the patient disagree as to the merits of abortion in a particular case.[24]

18 *Vö v France* [2004] ECHR 326, para. 82.
19 Plomer A. A foetal right to life? The case of *Vö v France. Human Rights Law Rev.* 2005; 5(2): 311–38.
20 *See Handyside v United Kingdom* (1976) 1 EHRR 737.
21 *Paton v United Kingdom* (1980) 3 EHRR 408, E Com HR.
22 *Glass v United Kingdom* [2004] ECHR 103.
23 *Brüggemann and Scheuten v Germany* (1981) 3 EHRR 244.
24 *Tysiac v Poland* [2007] ECHR 219.

13 Negligence before birth

13.1 INTRODUCTION

It is possible for negligence to occur before the birth of a child. The legal actions considered here differ from those considered elsewhere because they rest on the following premises:

(i)   the child was born alive

(ii) the negligence occurred before the child was born, and

(iii) the negligence in some way resulted in a harm suffered by the child.

There are broadly two types of complaint that can be made. A complaint of negligence can be made if:

(i)   The child is born injured. If the child is born healthy then no damage has arisen and therefore the action for negligent breach of duty fails for want of damage (*see* Section 8)

(ii) The child was born but should not have been born. Note that if the wrongful act causes the death of the fetus different rules apply (*see* Section 12.1.1). Also, if this is the claim, then the child can be born healthy.

In essence, the structure of the claim in negligence follows the usual principles (*see* Sections 8–11). But this structure is distorted slightly because questions of moral value surround the fetus. It is wise to be acquainted with the general principles of negligence before venturing into this modified variant. The main superadded issues are:

(i)   The negligence affects at least two people, the mother and the child.

Thus there are two sources of action to consider. The character of the legal actions available to each differs. The possibility that they may sue each other is legally restricted on grounds of public policy[1] (*see* Section 13.3.14).

---

1   s 1(1) *Congenital Disabilities (Civil Liability) Act 1976.*

(ii) The fact that the fetus is not a legal person (*see* Section 12).

We have already seen that whilst a fetus is recognised by law and has legal protections it cannot sustain a legal action because it lacks full legal personality.[2] Therefore, it cannot sustain a legal action until it is born alive.

(ii) Assessment of the value of non-existence can enter the considerations.

In a negligence action, once breach of the duty of care has been established, we are driven to compare what would have happened if the negligence had not occurred with what actually did happen. Because we are considering a fetus it can sometimes become necessary to weigh the life of the child that fetus has become against the hypothetical but imponderable alternative that the child was never born.

(iii) The possibility of abortion also resides implicitly within this legal structure.

This arises when the mother of a child had or should have had the option of an abortion after the negligence arose. For example, there is the argument that, where possible, the person suffering harm should act to reduce the harm that they have suffered. Their claim for damages cannot, therefore, include harm that flows from the negligence but which could have been prevented. The general principle here is that, despite this argument, it is not unlawful for the parents to choose to keep a child by refusing abortion or adoption.[3,4] Conversely, if a mother chooses to accept a lawful abortion then she cannot be prevented from a undergoing it by a third party[5] (*see* Section 14.2.1).

13.2 BUT FOR THE NEGLIGENCE THE CHILD WOULD NOT HAVE BEEN BORN AT ALL

13.2.1 Where the child, but for the negligence, would not have been born the harm in law is the existence of the child. It is important to note that the issue here is not about whether the child is born healthy or

---

2 *A-G's Reference (No.3 of 1994)* [1997] 3 All ER 936.
3 *Emeh v Kensington and Chelsea and Westminster Area Health Authority* [1984] 3 All ER 1044, 1053 per Slade LJ.
4 *McFarlane v Tayside Health Board* [1999] 4 All ER 961 at 970, 976, 990, 998, 1004 per Slynn Ld, Steyn Ld, Hope Ld, Clyde Ld and Millett Ld, respectively.
5 *C v S* [1987] 1 All ER 1230.

not. This claim might arise where the parents sought contraception, medical or surgical, and this failed. It might also arise where the child was conceived but was born in the face of a negligently performed abortion.[6]

13.2.2 Because prenatal breach affects two people, the mother and the child, we must consider the actions available to each under each consequence. The two claims are:

(1) Wrongful life – Child: 'I should never have been born'

(2) Wrongful conception – Parents: 'I should not have conceived this child.'

[1] The child's claim: 'I should never have been born.'

13.2.3 *McKay v Essex AHA*[7] was a rare case where the value of life, death and non-existence all fell to be considered together. The negligence here was a failure to diagnose prenatal rubella. The injury to the child was inflicted by the rubella virus not D. Thus the claim against D was not for allowing the child to suffer disability but for allowing the child to exist with the disability. This, in fact, reduced to a claim that the child should not have been allowed to exist at all. It was this last claim that was found to lack foundation.

McKay v Essex AHA [1982] 2 All ER 771, CA

P was a 6½-year-old girl who had suffered *in utero* rubella infection during the first trimester. As a result of the infection P was born severely disabled. She was congenitally partially sighted and partially deaf, and had other disabilities as a result of the infection. However, her life was not so awful or intolerable that it should be ended.[8]

P's mother had been attended by D who knew that she had had a recent infection. D discovered but negligently failed to tell P's mother that she had had rubella and that this would place P at risk of significant disability. It was pleaded that had P's mother known these facts she would have accepted a lawful abortion.

P sued for wrongful life and prenatal negligence. D sought to strike out the claims as disclosing no cause of action.

---

6   *Allen v Bloomsbury Health Authority* [1993] 1 All ER 651.
7   [1982] 2 All ER 771.
8   *Re: B (a minor) (wardship: medical treatment)* (1981) [1990] 3 All ER 927, para. 19.12.1.

Held: Action struck out.

The injury to P was caused by the rubella not the doctor's negligence.[9] Therefore, P could only rely on the claim that she should not have been born. The Court was unanimous that there was no action available for wrongful life.[10]

13.2.4   The child's claim for wrongful birth fails for a number of reasons:

(i)   The problem is that the child must argue that non-existence is preferable to life. But the value of non-existence cannot be determined, and so it cannot be compared with the value of the life to the child. This makes it impossible for any damage to be established even for a child born disabled.

(ii)   The child must claim that the duty that was breached by D was a duty to terminate its life. This claim rests on a fetal interest in dying. But the fetus lacks a legal persona and, in any case, the recognition of a claim based upon an interest in dying is contrary to legal policy and the principle of the sanctity of life[11] (*see* Section 19.4.4).

(iii)   If the child's claim to not be born carried force, then a fetal claim would operate to invade the mother's choices in relation to abortion.[12] Whilst there may be a duty owed to the mother to inform her of the extent of her child's disabilities and that abortion would be a lawful option, D owes no such duty to the child.[13] Even if the mother is offered lawful abortion there is no duty upon the mother to accept such an offer.[14] The fact that the mother was willing to undergo abortion had she been aware of the child's disability did not relieve the fact that the claim riled against legal policy and the principle of the sanctity of life.

13.2.5   Where the child born is so severely disabled that it could be argued their life was not worth living, a case for wrongful birth might appear

---

9   Although the general damages option used in *Rees v Darlington Memorial Hospital NHS Trust* [2003] 4 All ER 987, [2003] UKHL 52 might be apposite on similar facts given that the negligence removed a choice that the mother would have had in relation to possibility of abortion.

10   *See*, also, para. 89 Law Commission's Report on Injuries to Unborn Children (Law Com no 60, August 1974; Cmnd 5709).

11   *McKay v Essex AHA* [1982] 2 All ER 771, 786 per Ackner LJ.

12   *McKay v Essex AHA* [1982] 2 All ER 771, 786 per Ackner LJ.

13   *McKay v Essex AHA* [1982] 2 All ER 771, 780 per Stephenson LJ.

14   *McKay v Essex AHA* [1982] 2 All ER 771, 780 per Stephenson LJ.

to be arguable.[15,16] However here the comparison would be with death rather than non-existence. A healthy child arguing such a case faces an insurmountable barrier.[17]

[2] The parents' claim: 'I should not have conceived this child.'

13.2.6 From the perspective of the mother and father, the negligence has resulted in the birth of an unwanted, albeit healthy, child. The undesired pregnancy imposes physical costs upon the mother. The existence of an additional child in the household also imposes additional financial costs upon the household including food, clothing and schooling.

13.2.7 We have seen that negligence classifies harm into several types making some easier to recover than others (*see* Sections 9.5 and 9.7). This reflects the nature of the action. It grants more protection to physical harm than to other types of harm.[18] Therefore, the question of how to classify each type of harm is important.

13.2.8 For the purposes of negligence pregnancy is classified as a type of physical injury[19] (*see* para. 9.5.2). Despite pregnancy being generally regarded as a natural process,[20] it is not without risk of hazard. This categorisation makes it possible to justify the recovery of damages for the actual pregnancy and the consequent financial losses flowing directly from the pregnancy.[21,22]

13.2.9 Distinct from the economic costs flowing directly from the pregnancy itself are the costs of bringing up the child. Note that for these costs no rational distinction can be made between the claim of a father and that of a mother.[23] This contrasts with the economic costs flowing directly from the pregnancy.

13.2.10 A series of cases in the lower courts over a period of 15 years caused a degree of confusion about whether these costs could be recovered. In 1999 the House of Lords finally addressed the question and decided against permitting recovery.

---

15   *McKay v Essex AHA* [1982] 2 All ER 771, 780 per Stephenson LJ.
16   *McKay v Essex AHA* [1982] 2 All ER 771, 789 per Griffiths LJ.
17   *Zapeda v Zepeda* (1963) 190 NE 2d 849, Ill App Ct.
18   para. 56 *Parkinson v St James and Seacroft University Hospital NHS Trust* [2001] EWCA Civ 530, [2001] 3 All ER 97 per Hale LJ.
19   *Walkin v South Manchester HA* [1995] 4 All ER 132.
20   *McFarlane v Tayside Health Board* [1999] 4 All ER 961, 976 per Steyn Ld.
21   *McFarlane v Tayside Health Board* [1999] 4 All ER 961.
22   para. 68 *Parkinson v St James and Seacroft University Hospital NHS Trust* [2001] EWCA Civ 530, [2001] 3 All ER 97 per Hale LJ.
23   *McFarlane v Tayside Health Board* [1999] 4 All ER 961, 975 per Steyn Ld.

13.2.11 In the next few paragraphs we will briefly overview some of the earlier cases before examining the leading House of Lords case in more detail. The point to take from the brief overview of the earlier cases is an idea of how the common law evolves.

13.2.12 In 1983 a Court of first instance held that the costs of bringing up a healthy child were not recoverable.[24] In the following year another case at first instance on similar facts resulted in the opposite conclusion.[25] A subsequent decision by the Court of Appeal reviewed these conflicting positions and permitted recovery of the costs of bringing up a healthy child.[26] This decision of the Court of Appeal decision-bound future decisions of the lower courts of first instance and future decisions of the Court of Appeal itself.

13.2.13 A general approach developed such that, provided causation could be established,[27] the costs of bringing up a healthy child until adulthood could be recovered in cases of wrongful conception.[28,29,30] Indeed this principle extended to permit recovery of the future cost of a private education for the child in one case.[31]

13.2.14 In 1999 a fresh case finally reached the House of Lords. The House of Lords is not bound by the decisions of the lower courts. Its view was that the costs of bringing up a healthy but initially unwanted child were **not** recoverable.

13.2.15 The essential legal issue here is that, but for the negligence, there would have been no child. A wrong has been committed. The costs of rearing a child are a foreseeable consequence of this negligence. The costs of bringing up a child flow inexorably from the negligence and in principle should be recoverable. Yet, by a majority, the House of Lords denied recovery.

---

24   *Udale v Bloomsbury AHA* [1983] 2 All ER 522, QBD.
25   *Thake v Maurice* [1984] 2 All ER 513 which permitted recovery of the cost of bringing up a healthy child, but not the costs associated with the pain and suffering of the unwanted pregnancy.
26   *Emeh v Kensington and Chelsea and Westminster Area Health Authority* [1984] 3 All ER 1044, CA.
27   *Salih v Enfield Health Authority* [1991] 3 All ER 400.
28   *Allen v Bloomsbury Health Authority* [1993] 1 All ER 651.
29   *Crouchman v Burke* (1997) 40 BMLR 163.
30   *Robinson v Salford Health Authority* [1992] 3 Med LR 270.
31   *Benarr v Kettering Health Authority* (1988) 138 NLJ 179.

McFarlane v Tayside Health Board [1999] 4 All ER 961[32]

Slynn Ld, Steyn Ld, Hope Ld, Clyde Ld and Millett Ld

P and W were married with four children. P underwent a vasectomy in order to limit the size of their family. After six months P was told his sperm counts were negative and that he could have unprotected intercourse. P and W relied on this advice. W became pregnant giving birth to a healthy daughter.

P and W sued. The claim was for £10 000 for the pain and suffering attributable to the pregnancy and a further £100 000 for the cost of bringing up the child.

Held: Could recover for the physical harm of the pregnancy and its associated economic loss, but could not recover for the costs of rearing a healthy child. There is no duty upon the parents to reduce their financial loss by considering abortion or surrendering the child for adoption.

Ld Steyn: Rejected recovery for the costs of bringing up the child on the basis of an 'an inarticulate premise as to what is morally acceptable and what is not'. This amounted to a value judgement that a healthy child is a good thing and an appeal to the principle of distributive justice.[33]

Ld Slynn and Hope: Regarded the costs of bringing up a healthy child as purely economic loss. The duty owed extended to cover the physical harm of pregnancy and its consequent costs but not to the economic loss of bringing up the child.

Ld Millett: Regarded the distinction between pure economic loss and financial loss related to the physical injury as 'technical and artificial'.[34] He accepted a moral distaste in allowing recovery of damages for the birth of a healthy child and refused the claim for the costs of bringing up the healthy child on the basis that the child was a blessing not a detriment.

Ld Clyde: Took a completely different path. He looked to the extent that might be recovered once negligence had been established. He felt that it was unreasonable[35] to allow the recovery of the costs of bringing up the child given a lack of proportionality between the wrongdoing and the extent of the liability. Reflecting that the doctors were unlikely to have considered that they were undertaking a liability to provide for the full costs of bringing up a child he concluded that the costs of bringing up the healthy child were not recoverable.

---

32 Followed in *AD v East Kent Community NHS Trust* [2003] 3 All ER 1167 [2002] EWCA Civ 1872.
33 *McFarlane v Tayside Health Board* [1999] 4 All ER 961, 976 per Steyn Ld.
34 *McFarlane v Tayside Health Board* [1999] 4 All ER 961, 1000.
35 *Allan v Greater Glasgow Health Board* (1993) 1998 SLT 580 at 585.

Ld Millett: Agreed that the costs of rearing a child should not be recoverable, but dissented in refusing P recovery for the physical harm of the pregnancy, replacing this with a sum given to P and W for general damages. In addition to the damages for pain and suffering Ld Millett would have granted a sum of general damages for the reduction in autonomy in relation to their life choices imposed by the presence of an additional child (see, also, Section 13.3.20).[36]

13.2.16 Looking for grounds to deny recovery of these costs there are, broadly, two powerful arguments:

(i) One can view the costs that flow directly from the pregnancy as differing in character from the costs of bringing up the child: the former being physical injury whilst the latter might be seen as purely economic loss. Pure economic loss is easier to recover where it flows from a breach of contract than when it flows from negligence in the absence of a contract. But even where the action is for breach of contract, the Court is slow to find that a doctor implicitly guarantees the success of a particular treatment[37]

(ii) One can argue that what the surgeon undertook to achieve was a treatment that was aimed at preventing pregnancy. On this view the surgeon did not guarantee to succeed, only to exercise due skill and care when undertaking the procedure.

13.2.17 It has been noted that the deep principle underlying these lines of reasoning is that it is not fair, just and reasonable to permit recovery for the costs of bringing up a healthy child in cases of wrongful conception.[38,39] The legal policy arguments were subsequently crystallised[40] as being:

(i) a refusal to see a child as only a financial burden (the value of a child could not be calculated)

(ii) a recognition of the impossibility of quantifying the rewards of (involuntary) parenthood, and

---

36 para. 124 *Rees v Darlington Memorial Hospital NHS Trust* [2003] 4 All ER 987.
37 *Eyre v Measday* [1986] 1 All ER 488, CA; *Thake v Maurice* [1986] 1 All ER 497, CA.
38 para. 85 *Rees v Darlington Memorial Hospital NHS Trust* [2003] 4 All ER 987 per Hutton Ld.
39 para. 106 *Rees v Darlington Memorial Hospital NHS Trust* [2003] 4 All ER 987 per Millett Ld.
40 para. 6 *Rees v Darlington Memorial Hospital NHS Trust* [2003] 4 All ER 987 per Bingham Ld.

(iii) the discomfort to the principle of distributive justice caused by requiring a cash-strapped NHS to pay potentially very large sums of public money to the parents of healthy children.

13.2.18 The direct costs to the mother of the pregnancy, including pain and suffering, were recoverable in *McFarlane v Tayside Health Board*[41] because the claim by the mother is one for personal injury not economic loss.[42] For a pregnancy to amount to harm it should be unwanted.[43]

Walkin v South Manchester HA **[1995] 4 All ER 132, CA**

P sought sterilisation for financial reasons. D negligently performed sterilisation by laparoscopic tubal diathermy. P became pregnant afterwards. P sued for wrongful conception: failure to inform of risk of failure and negligently performed procedure. The claim for personal injury was statute barred but P claimed economic loss recovery which was not statute barred.

It was contended on behalf of P that personal injury action arises from the pregnancy, but that there is also a separate right not to be subjected to the financial burdens of parenthood that could give rise to an independent claim for economic loss.

Held: Damages flowed from the pregnancy which fell within the meaning of 'impairment' in s 38(1) Limitation Act 1980. The action was thus one for personal injury within the terms of the Limitation Act 1980 and was statute barred.

13.3 BUT FOR THE NEGLIGENCE THE CHILD WOULD NOT HAVE BEEN BORN DISABLED

13.3.1 The basic complaint here is that but for the negligence the child would not have been injured in some way. The key distinguishing point for this class of cases is that there is a necessary connection between the negligence and the child's disability.[44]

---

41 *McFarlane v Tayside Health Board* [1999] 4 All ER 961.
42 *See* also *Greenfield v Flather* [2001] EWCA Civ 113 where loss of earnings was not recoverable as economic loss.
43 *Walkin v South Manchester HA* [1995] 4 All ER 132, 141 per Roche; *R v Croyden* (1990) 40 BMLR 40, 47 per Kennedy LJ.
44 *Groom v Selby* [2001] EWCA Civ 1522, para. 29 per Hale LJ.

13.3.2 This separates this class of cases from cases of wrongful conception where the negligence is causally linked to the birth of the child but not necessarily to any disability the child might suffer.

13.3.3 Because the prenatal breach affects two people, the mother and the child we must consider the actions available to each under each consequence. The two claims are:
(1) Prenatal negligence – Child: 'I should not have suffered this disability'
(2) Wrongful birth – Parents: 'Our child should not be injured.'

(3) The child's claim: 'I should not have suffered this disability.'

13.3.4 The child complains that but for the negligence occurring before they were born they would not have suffered physical injury. The difficulties to constructing this action are based in the fact that at the time the negligence occurred the child was not yet born and therefore lacked full legal personality (*see* Section 12). The respondent can argue that:

(i) their negligence did not breach any duty owed to any legal person

(ii) their negligence did not harm any legal person, and/or

(iii) that the harm suffered by the child once born was not causally linked to their negligence.

(a) Case law

13.3.5 The case law has been replaced by the *Congenital Disabilities (Civil Liability) Act 1976* for children born since 21 July 1976 (*see* Section 13.3.9).[45] We will consider briefly the common law position to make a point (*see* Section 13.3.8) about the logic underpinning the theoretical structure that gave rise to the present position under the *Congenital Disabilities (Civil Liability) Act 1976*.

13.3.6 The view taken in the following case was that once the negligent breach of duty had occurred then the action of negligence did not crystallise until the injured child was born. However, once the injured child was born, provided its physical injury could be causally related to the negligence, then an action for negligence would lie at the suit of the child.

---

45   s 4(5) *Congenital Disabilities (Civil Liability) Act 1976.*

Watt v Rama [1972] VR 353, full court of Supreme Court of Victoria[46]

Winneke CJ, Pape, Gillard JJ

Negligent driving led to a road accident involving a pregnant woman. P was a child who was subsequently born suffering from brain damage, epilepsy and tetraplegia. In order to address the issues causation was assumed by the Court.

Held: The child (P) could maintain an action for prenatal injury.

All three judges accepted that there was no reason why the breach of duty and the damage suffered by P could not be separated in time. There were two broad views of how this separation of the breach of duty and the damage suffered could be separated in time:

Winneke CJ and Pape J: The duty of care was contingent. Where it was breached the negligence action crystallised when the damage was suffered by a legal person, i.e. when the injured child was born.

Gillard J: The fetus had a right of action but could not exercise that right until it had legal personality, i.e. until it was born.

13.3.7   This Australian case was followed by the English Court of Appeal when it dealt with the same issue.

Burton v Islington HA, de Martell v Merton and Sutton HA [1992] 3 All ER 833, CA

Dillon, Balcombe and Leggatt LJJ

Two cases were heard together by the Court of Appeal on a single point of law.

Burton v Islington H: Plaintiff's mother was five weeks pregnant. Mother underwent a dilatation and curettage (D&C). The defendant negligently failed to perform a pregnancy test prior to the procedure. The plaintiff was born with deformed limbs and an inability to conceive.

Potts J: At first instance preferred reasoning of Winneke CJ and Pape J in *Watt v Rama*.

de Martell v Merton and Sutton HA: Plaintiff suffered for injuries due to negligent delivery.

Phillips J: At first instance preferred reasoning of Gillard J (duty in existence and breached at time of insult) in *Watt v Rama*.

---

46   *See*, also, *Duval v Seguin* (1972) 26 DLR (3d) 418, High Court Ontario.

Held: There was a right of action for prenatal injury at the suit of a child born alive.

Dillon LJ: There was no need to distinguish between the two lines of reasoning in *Watt v Rama* since both lead to the same conclusion.

Balcombe and Leggatt LJJ: Agreed.

13.3.8 Duties can only be owed to those with legal persona. A breach of a duty can only occur if the duty exists. However, it is not until birth that the child gains a full legal persona. Therefore the common law action is founded upon a breach of a duty *owed to the injured child*. The gap in time between the act of negligence and the crystallisation of the action combining both a breach of duty and damage is bridged by a (fictional) legal suspension of the claim until the birth of the child. Whether you regard this as a suspension of the breach or a crystallisation of the harm does not change the conclusion.

(b) Congenital Disabilities (Civil Liability) Act 1976

13.3.9 Another, but different, solution to the same problem is provided by the *Congenital Disabilities (Civil Liability) Act 1976* as amended *(CD(CL) A 1976)*. This has been available since 21 July 1976.[47] It replaces the common law from this date. The mechanism of this claim is to take the rights associated with a breach of a duty owed by D to one of the parents of a child and transfer them to the child once they are born alive. Once the child is born alive, the magic of the statute unites the breach against the parents and the injuries suffered by the child creating a right of action in favour of the child.[48]

13.3.10 The elegance of this claim is that it only requires the existence of duties that arise between existing legal personae. Thus the fetal lack of legal persona does not defeat the claim. Conversely the fetal claim only crystallises when the child is born alive. The damage is deemed to arise at birth.[49] This makes the claim one for personal injury as though suffered after birth by the child.[49]

13.3.11 There are, of course, constraints on the claim. The *CD(CL)A 1976* provides that D (a person other than the mother) must cause an

---

47   s 4(5) *Congenital Disabilities (Civil Liability) Act 1976.*
48   s 1(1) and s 4(2)(a) *Congenital Disabilities (Civil Liability) Act 1976.*
49   s 4(3) *Congenital Disabilities (Civil Liability) Act 1976.*

'occurrence' before the birth of the child. The person harmed and the requisite harm to trigger the provisions is set out in **Table 3**.

TABLE 3 Congenital Disabilities (Civil Liability) Act 1976 – requisite harms and persons affected.

Provision	Effects	Resulting in
s 2(a) CD(CL)A 1976	Either or both parents	Affecting the ability to have a normal child
s 2(b) CD(CL)A 1976	Mother during pregnancy, or mother or child during childbirth	A child born with disabilities

13.3.12 D must be liable to the affected parent for the breach of a duty in tort.[50] This claim extends to harm flowing from infertility treatments, including the selection and keeping or use of embryos or gametes outside the body.[51] Where D is delivering professional services then regard must be had to received professional opinion when determining whether D acted with due care.[50]

13.3.13 Because the claim is derivative from the breach of the duty of care owed to the parents, the child's claim is subject to any defences that D possesses against the parental claim.[52] These include contractual exemption clauses[53] and any contributory negligence on the part of the affected parent.[53] The child's claim is also limited where the parents had knowledge of the risk that materialised. The knowledge must be possessed by the mother alone or by both parents.[54,55]

13.3.14 For policy reasons the child cannot sue their own mother.[56]

(4) The parents' claim: 'Our child should not be injured.'

13.3.15 Where the claim is that the child should not have been born with disabilities then it is still possible for the parents to recover for the costs they incur for the child's disability which flow from the negligent breach.[57] Whilst they cannot recover for the costs of a healthy child,[58]

---

50   s 1(5) *Congenital Disabilities (Civil Liability) Act 1976.*
51   s 1A *Congenital Disabilities (Civil Liability) Act 1976.*
52   s 1(6) *Congenital Disabilities (Civil Liability) Act 1976.*
53   s 1(7) *Congenital Disabilities (Civil Liability) Act 1976.*
54   s 1(4) *Congenital Disabilities (Civil Liability) Act 1976.*
55   para. 93 Law Commission's Report on Injuries to Unborn Children (Law Com no. 60, August 1974; Cmnd 5709).
56   s 1(1) *Congenital Disabilities (Civil Liability) Act 1976.*
57   *Rand v East Dorset Health Authority* [2000] Lloyd's Rep Med 181; *Farraj v King's Healthcare NHS Trust* [2006] EWHC 1228.
58   *Greenfield v Irwin (A Firm)* [2001] EWCA Civ 113.

they can recover for the disabilities on the basis that the costs of bringing up a disabled child are greater than the corresponding costs of bringing up a healthy child.

13.3.16   Looking at this claim from the child's perspective, the disability could have been directly caused by D's negligence in which case the child may have a claim under the *Congenital Disabilities (Civil Liability) Act 1976* as amended.

13.3.17   Alternatively, it could be that the disability was caused by another agent but that D failed to diagnose the condition. In this situation the child's parents would have lost the opportunity to choose abortion or accept treatment that might have ameliorated or relieved the disability. Here the child cannot claim wrongful life (*see* Section 13.2).

13.3.18   In either scenario the parents can argue that they must bear the costs of the child's disability which would not have arisen had there not been negligence. The principles for wrongful birth and wrongful conception are the same.[59]

Parkinson v St James and Seacroft University Hospital NHS Trust [2001] EWCA Civ 530, CA

P was the mother of four children. She sought sterilisation by tubal ligation. D performed a negligent laparoscopic sterilisation upon P, failing to occlude the left fallopian tube. In addition, two Filshie clips found their way into P's Pouch of Douglas. P subsequently underwent laparotomy with salpingectomy.

P became pregnant and delivered a child who had an autistic spectrum disorder with special needs. P sued, inter alia, for the added costs of bringing up the child that resulted from his disability.

Held: P could recover these additional costs.

The principle in *McFarlane v Tayside Health Board*[60] applied to healthy children. It could not be said that the issues of legal policy underpinning that decision also applied to the claim in this case.

To recover, the disability had to be something that resulted in substantial and permanent handicap.[61] The disability can arise after conception if it is a foreseeable risk of pregnancy (e.g. genetic disorders, rubella or prenatal hypoxia).

---

59   *Groom v Selby* [2001] EWCA Civ 1522, para. 28 per Hale LJ.
60   [1999] 4 All ER 961.
61   *Parkinson v St James and Seacroft University Hospital NHS Trust* [2001] EWCA Civ 530, para. 91 per Hale LJ referring to ss 17(10) and 17(11) *Children Act 1989*.

13.3.19 Where a healthy child is born to a disabled parent, the disabled parent cannot recover for the additional costs of bringing up a child that flows from the parent's disability. A seven-judge-strong Court (normally five judges in the House of Lords) convened to consider whether to reverse their previous decision in *McFarlane v Tayside Health Board*.[62] After careful consideration, but only by a bare majority of 4:3, they felt that the decision in *McFarlane* was right and should not be reversed. The area is clearly contentious with other jurisdictions permitting recovery.[63]

Rees v Darlington Memorial Hospital NHS Trust [2003] UKHL 52, [2003] 4 All ER 987, HL

Bingham Ld, Nicholls Ld, Steyn Ld, Hope Ld, Hutton Ld, Millett Ld, Scott Ld

P suffered from retinitis pigmentosa and was registered partially sighted. She was blind in one eye with a visual acuity of 6/36 in the other eye. Her vision had been deteriorating further. She sought sterilisation in order to ensure that she was not forced to take on the responsibilities of looking after a child. These were responsibilities she felt she could not cope with because of her disability.

D performed a negligent sterilisation procedure, failing to occlude the right fallopian tube. P subsequently gave birth to a healthy child.

P sought to recover the additional costs of bringing up the child that were consequent to P's disability.

Held (4:3): P could not recover for the costs of bringing up the child.

P's disability was not caused by D. P could not recover on the basis of the reasoning in *McFarlane v Tayside Health Board*,[64] a decision which should not be reversed. The majority were also swayed by possibility that social and economic disability could found similar claims.[65] In some cases, this might lead to a perception that the principle of distributive justice had been breached.

In addition to P's claim for pain and suffering arising from the pregnancy itself, the House awarded a sum of £15000 for the breach of her autonomy

---

62 [1999] 4 All ER 961.
63 *Cattanach v Melchior* [2003] HCA 38, Sup Ct Australia; *Lovelace Medical Center v Mendez* (1991) 805 P 2d 603, New Mexico.
64 [1999] 4 All ER 961.
65 *Rees v Darlington Memorial Hospital NHS Trust* [2002] EWCA Civ 88, CA paras. 53–55 per Waller LJ.

caused by the negligence. This was based on the reasoning of Slynn Ld in *McFarlane v Tayside Health Board*[66] (*see* Section 13.2.14).

13.3.20 Where the cause of the harm is operating at the time of the crystallisation of the negligence, even if the damage has not yet occurred, then recovery may still be possible. This is a causation point but arises in this context in the following case.

Groom v Selby [2001] EWCA Civ 1522, CA

D was a GP who failed to diagnose P was pregnant after a competent sterilisation operation. It was likely that P had conceived just before the sterilisation. P gave birth to a child three weeks prematurely. The child was born healthy but developed salmonella meningitis at three weeks. This was complicated by bilateral frontal lobe abscesses with consequent disability.
  P sued for wrongful birth.

Held: P could recover.
  The negligence had been admitted. Although the child was born apparently healthy, it was found that it harboured the salmonella bacterium from its birth. The causal chain between the negligence and the meningitis was not broken and P could recover.

13.3.21 The amount recovered may reflect a continuing burden upon the parents after the child reaches adulthood.[67] It may also reflect the fact that the parents would have had another child even if they would have chosen abortion in the immediate case in the absence of negligence.

Salidh v Enfield HA [1991] 3 All ER 400, CA

D failed to diagnose prenatal rubella resulting in the birth of a severely handicapped child suffering from congenital rubella syndrome. P lost the opportunity to consider termination. If the pregnancy had been terminated, then the parents would have had another (presumably healthy) child.

---

66 [1999] 4 All ER 961, 1005.
67 *Nunnerley v Warrington Health Authority* [2000] Lloyd's Rep Med 170 – defective genetic counselling. Parents entitled to full upkeep of child until and after 18th birthday. Also *Taylor v Shropshire Health Authority* [2000] Lloyd's Rep Med 96 (QBD).

Held: Could recover the additional costs of the disability.

The general costs of maintaining a child would have been incurred in any case because the parents would have had another (presumably healthy) child in the event of termination.

13.4 CONCLUSION

13.4.1 The child lacks a wrongful life claim but, by virtue of the *Congenital Disabilities (Civil Liability) Act 1976* as amended, possesses a claim for prenatal negligence despite lacking a legal personality when the breach of duty occurred.

13.4.2 The parents can claim for wrongful conception and the consequent losses as personal injury. They can also claim for the additional costs of bringing up a disabled child as part of a wrongful birth claim. However they cannot recover the costs of bringing up a healthy child.

13.4.3 There is no obligation to undergo abortion.

14 Abortion

14.1 FUNDAMENTAL PRINCIPLES

14.1.1 Abortion is the deliberate termination of pregnancy. The outcome is the loss of the fetus. This is an emotive and often divisive issue. The structure of law in this area is one of a blanket of criminal sanction with areas of lawfulness. Thus it is a criminal offence to procure or perform an abortion. Section 58 of the *Offences Against the Person Act 1861* makes it unlawful for anyone, including the pregnant woman, to procure a miscarriage (*see* paras. 12.1.5–12.1.10)

14.1.2 In 1938 the breadth of the exception to this crime of child destruction was tested.

R v Bourne [1938] 3 All ER 615 (CCC)

V was a 14-year-old girl who had become pregnant after being raped. A man had been convicted for the rape. D was a gynaecologist of good standing who openly undertook the abortion in hospital. He charged no fee.

D was charged with procuring an abortion unlawfully under section 58 of the *Offences Against the Person Act 1861*.

In the direction to jury, McNaughten J distinguished these facts from a backstreet abortion type case. He interpreted the word 'unlawfully' in section 58 of the *Offences Against the Person Act 1861* as importing the exception found in the offence of child destruction created by the *Infant Life (Preservation) Act 1929*. This meant that the word 'unlawfully' implied that '. . . the act which caused the death of the child was not done in good faith for the purpose only of preserving the life of the mother.'.

He then held that a 'reasonable' view needed to be taken of the words 'for the purpose of preserving the life of the mother'. Such a view could incorporate the likelihood that continuance of the pregnancy would make the woman 'a physical or mental wreck'.

Jury verdict: D acquitted.

14.1.3   The effect of the *Bourne* case was to expand the justifications for lawful abortion from a threat to the life of the mother to include significant threats to the mental and physical health of the mother.

14.1.4   After a period of political and social debate the justifications for lawful abortion[1] were expanded further by the introduction of the *Abortion Act 1967*. This created five broad lawful justifications for abortion (*see* **Table 4**). Essentially the justifications cover:

  (i)   threat to the life of the pregnant woman

  (ii) threat to her physical or mental health

  (iii) threat of severe disability to the fetus if born, and

  (iv) as an extension to principle, threat to the mental or physical health of the pregnant mother's existing children.

    One of these interests must be threatened both to an extent and to a degree of certainty as defined in the Act. (*see* **Table 4**, p. 171).

14.1.5   Early abortion is justified on a broader range of grounds than later abortion to reflect the increasing claim that the fetus has as it develops. The justifications do extend to cover late abortion albeit with more restrictive grounds. These late grounds encompass significant risk of harm to the mother or fetus if delivered. Notice that the effects upon the mother's other children is not justification for late abortion.

14.1.6   In multiple pregnancies, which became more common with the increasing use of reproductive technology, selective abortions were made lawful by an amendment to the *Abortion Act 1967* made by section 37 of the *Human Fertilisation and Embryology Act 1990*.

---

1   s 1(1) *Abortion Act 1967*; s 5(1) *Abortion Act 1967* as amended by s 37 *Human Fertilisation Act 1990*.

TABLE 4 Grounds for lawful termination under the Abortion Act 1967 as amended.[2]

Subsection	Time limit	Risk of injury to whom?	Risk of what injury?	How much risk of that injury?	How severe must the injury be?	Consider actual or reasonably foreseeable environment of pregnant woman?[3]
s 1(1)(a)	24 weeks gestation or less	i) Pregnant woman ii) Existing children of pregnant woman's family	Injury to mental or physical health	Risk of injury greater with continuation of pregnancy than if terminate pregnancy[4]		Yes
s 1(1)(b)	No time limit	Pregnant woman	Injury to mental or physical health	Termination is 'necessary'[5]	Potential grave permanent injury[6]	Yes
s 1(1)(c)[7]	No time limit	Pregnant woman	Loss of life[8] of pregnant woman	Risk of injury greater with continuation of pregnancy than if pregnancy terminated.	Potential death of pregnant woman	No
s 1(1)(d)	No time limit	Child, if born	Mental or physical abnormalities such as to be seriously handicapped	Substantial risk[9]	Potential serious handicap[10]	No
s 1(4) Emergency (two doctors not required)	No time limit	Pregnant woman	i) Loss of life, or ii) injury to mental or physical health	Termination is immediately 'necessary'[5]	i) Loss of life, or ii) potential grave permanent injury	No

2 s 37 *Human Fertilisation and Embryology Act 1990*. Amendments to the *Abortion Act 1967* made by s 37 *HFEA 1990* came into operation on 1 April 1991.

3 s 1(2) *Abortion Act 1967*.

(Table 4 footnotes continued on folloiwng page.)

171

14.1.7   Except for the case of an emergency, two registered medical practitioners acting in good faith have to certify that these conditions have been met.[11] This creates a device that protects against misuse of the provisions, but the device does rest heavily upon professional integrity and professional values. In addition, the treatment must be provided in an NHS hospital or other approved place.[12] (These additional two requirements do not apply to the emergency exception under section 1(4).)

14.1.8   How the legal structure in this area impacts upon medical care is made apparent by **Table 5**. Most abortions were performed to prevent injury to the mental and physical health of the pregnant woman, the ground first countenanced in *R v Bourne* (*see* Section 14.1.1). As a result of the time limit set by this section, most abortions were performed early in pregnancy, with 68% of abortions performed under 10 weeks gestation and 22% between 10–12 weeks.

---

4   Unclear if this means greater risk of the same magnitude of injury. Alternatively, it could mean: risk of injury = Σ (probability of harm × magnitude of harm). The risk of injury must be separately assessed for each of the two options, i.e. continuation of pregnancy and termination of pregnancy.

5   Presumably 'necessary' means that the intervention will make it at least likely that the pregnant woman will avoid the nature and degree of injury defined as sufficient justification by the Act.

6   Excludes transient conditions that do not affect the pregnant woman's life. However, likely to cover postpartum dilated cardiomyopathy.

7   *See* Wicks E, Wyldes M, Kilby M. Late termination of pregnancy for fetal abnormality: medical and legal perspectives. *Med Law Rev.* 2004; **3**: 285–305.

8   Note the broad interpretation in *R v Bourne* [1938]3 All ER 615 – here must be defined narrowly because s 1(1)(a) and s 1(1)(b) exist.

9   per AJC Hoggett in The *Abortion Act 1967* [1968] Crim LR 247 'test should be – could any reasonable doctor consider this a substantial risk or a serious handicap?'

10   It does not cover mere possession of undesirable genes (e.g. cystic fibrosis), so it does not cover phenotypically normal carriers.

11   s 1(1) *Abortion Act 1967.*

12   s 1(3) *Abortion Act 1967.*

TABLE 5 Percentage of all lawful abortions performed by legal ground in England and Wales in 2006.[13]

Abortion Act 1967	Risk to whom	Risk of what?	% of total abortions in 2005
s 1(1)(a)	Pregnant woman	Injury to mental or physical health	96.9%
s 1(1)(a)	Existing children	Injury to mental or physical health	1.4%
s 1(1)(b)	Pregnant woman	Injury to mental or physical health	0.5%
s 1(1)(c)	Pregnant woman	Loss of life	0.1%
s 1(1)(d)	Child if born	Potential serious handicap	1.1%
s 1(4)	Pregnant woman	Loss of life	rare
s 1(4)	Pregnant woman	Injury to mental or physical health	

Total number of abortions in 2006: 193 737

14.1.9   In order to ensure that the necessary processes have been completed and to allow data collection, a legal requirement of certification exists. The opinion of the medical practitioners must be set out on a prescribed form[14] and notice of the procedure must be given to the Chief Medical Officer (CMO).[15] This disclosure is subject to a statutory obligation of confidentiality subject to exceptions that include notification of the CMO and the President of the GMC, as well as release of information for research purposes or to a senior police officer for the purpose of investigating a criminal offence, and to the practitioner undertaking the termination of pregnancy and other practitioners with the consent of the woman.[16]

14.1.10   The pregnancy must be terminated by a registered medical practitioner. This includes a situation where a doctor initiates the procedure but it is continued and completed in their absence by qualified nursing staff. Where the doctor prescribes the treatment, remains in charge and accepts responsibility throughout and the treatment is delivered in accordance with their direction the pregnancy is terminated by a medical practitioner within the terms of the *Abortion Act 1967*.[17]

---

13   Department of Health. Abortion Statistics, England and Wales: 2006.
14   Form HSA1.
15   *Abortion Regulations 1991* (SI 1991/499) as amended by *Abortion Regulations 2002* (SI 2002/887).
16   *Abortion Regulations 1991* (SI 1991/499), Regulation 5.
17   *Royal College of Nursing of the United Kingdom v Department of Health and Social Security* [1981] 1 All ER 54.

14.1.11 The medical practitioner must act in good faith. The burden is on the prosecution to prove beyond reasonable doubt that there was an absence of good faith. This is a difficult burden to discharge. In *R v Smith*[18] notice how, amongst other things, a failure to comply with the requirements of the Act permitted the jury to infer a lack of good faith.

R v Smith [1974] 1 All ER 376, CA

D undertook abortion on a 19-year-old girl. He received a fee of £150. The girl gave evidence that she had not seen a second medical professional.

At trial a second doctor gave evidence that they had given the required second medical opinion and had administered the anaesthetic during the procedure. The only evidence of assessment of mental health was in a note: 'mother knows: not willing to marry: depressed'.

The prosecution alleged that D had not made their decision in relation to the abortion in good faith.

A jury had convicted D of performing an unlawful abortion. A separate defence of merely tidying up after a spontaneous abortion was rejected by the jury. D appealed.

Held: Conviction upheld.

The question of good faith was one for the jury to determine.

14.1.12 There is no duty to participate in an abortion for those who have a **conscientious objection** to the procedure.[19] The duty is not removed in emergency circumstances where the life of the mother is at risk or the mother is at risk of suffering grave permanent injury to her mental or physical health. The person seeking to be released from the duty must demonstrate their conscientious objection.[20]

14.1.13 Participate means actually be involved in the procedure of the abortion. Thus a medical secretary who sought to rely on this provision to avoid having to type letters relating to abortions was found not to be participating in the procedures. She was, therefore, unable to take advantage of the provision.[21]

---

18   [1974] 1 All ER 376.
19   *McKay v Essex Area Health Authority* [1982] 2 All ER 771, 779 per Stephenson LJ.
20   s 4 *Abortion Act 1967*.
21   *Janaway v Salford HA* [1988] 3 All ER 1079, HL.

14.2 CONFLICTING INTERESTS

14.2.1 A father cannot prevent a pregnant mother from undergoing a lawful abortion.[22]

C v S [1987] 1 All ER 1230, CA

F and P were an unmarried couple. P was 18–21 weeks pregnant. F was the genetic father of P's child. P had established grounds for abortion under s 1(b) Abortion Act 1967.

F sought an injunction to prevent P seeking or obtaining a termination of pregnancy.

Held: Injunction not granted.

Termination of the pregnancy would not be unlawful. The Court declined to interfere with the discretion of the doctors under the Abortion Act 1967.

14.2.2 The facts were similar in *Paton v Trustees of BPAS*[23] except that the parents were married. The outcome was the same: the husband could not prevent his wife undergoing a lawful abortion. The abortion was carried out within hours of this decision. Despite this, the husband subsequently applied to the European Commission but, again, his application was unsuccessful.[24]

14.2.3 The interests of the fetus cannot be used to override the rights of the mother to be free from unjustified physical interference[25] (*see* Section 4.5.3). Because the fetus lacks legal status, the jurisdiction of the Court does not extend to exercising its powers over the mother to protect the fetal interests.

Re: F (in utero) [1988] Fam 122, CA

P was a 36-year-old pregnant woman who suffered from mental disturbance accompanied by drug abuse. She did not meet the criteria for treatment under the Mental Health Act 1983.

---

22 *See,* also, *H v Norway* (1992) 73 DR 155.
23 [1978] 2 All ER 987.
24 *Paton v United Kingdom* (1980) 3 EHRR 408, E Com HR.
25 *St Georges Healthcare NHS Trust v S* [1998] 3 All ER 673, CA; *Re: MB* (1997) 8 Med LR 217, CA.

The local authority sought to make the fetus a ward of court, thereby allowing the mother to be found and the medical interests of the fetus to be protected. The mother was not represented at the hearing.

Held: The Court had no power to make an unborn child a ward of court. It could not extend the law to impose control over the pregnant mother in order to benefit an unborn child.

14.3   CONCLUSION*

14.3.1   The basic structure is criminal liability with statutory exceptions. Note how most cases of abortion fall within s 1(1)(a) of the *Abortion Act 1967* as amended (*see* **Table 5**, p. 173).

---

*   This section could not include any changes that might arise from the presently proposed *Human Embryology and Fertilisation Bill 2008* (*see* para. 1.1.5).

15 Assisted reproduction

15.1 HUMAN FERTILISATION AND EMBRYOLOGY AUTHORITY

15.1.1   The provision of medically assisted reproduction is overseen by the Human Fertilisation and Embryology Authority (HFEA).[1] The HFEA is a government-appointed body with statutory powers that is charged with regulation of assisted reproduction services and the issuance of a code of practice in relation to those services. The HFEA was brought into existence by the *Human Fertilisation and Embryology Act 1990*.[2] This structure was recommended by the conclusions of the Warnock Committee which reported in 1984.[3]

15.1.2   Presently the HFEA remit includes storage of gametes; use of donor gametes or stored gametes but not the use of fresh sperm from a man treated together with a woman; *in vitro* fertilisation (IVF) including the use of micromanipulation techniques to create the embryo and special techniques to implant an embryo including zygote intrafallopian transfer (ZIFT); pre-implantation genetic screening, diagnosis and genetic haplotyping; and artificial insemination, including gamete intrafallopian transfer (GIFT), using donor gametes or stored sperm.

15.1.3   It can also license embryo research, but only until the development of the primitive streak or 14 days.[4] Other limits on permissible research include the use of embryos created other than by fertilisation (i.e. cloned embryos) for reproduction,[5,6] and the placing of a human

---

1   www.hfea.gov.uk.
2   The *Human Fertilisation and Embryology Act 1990* is likely to be subject to amendment by the *Human Tissues and Embryos Bill* which is under scrutiny by Parliament at the time of writing.
3   Warnock M (Chair). Report of the Committee of Enquiry into Human Fertilisation and Embryology. [1984] Cmnd.9314.
4   Schedule 2, para. 3 *Human Fertilisation and Embryology Act 1990*; *The Human Fertilisation and Embryology (Research Purposes) Regulations 2001*; part 10 HFEA Code of Practice 2003 (sixth edition, amended).
5   *R v Secretary of State for Health* ex parte *Quintavalle* [2003] UKHL 13, HL.
6   *Human Reproductive Cloning Act 2001*; s 3(3)(d) HFEA 1990.

embryo into an animal[7] – both of these are illegal. However, the mixing of human gametes with animal gametes can be made lawful by a licence from the HFEA.

15.1.4 The HFEA can regulate the provision of assisted reproduction services by issuing licences. It is a criminal offence to carry out regulated activities without a licence. The maximum penalty in certain situations is an unlimited fine or up to ten years imprisonment or both.[8,9] The licence conditions allow the HFEA to inspect the facilities providing the regulated services, require the licence holder to keep adequate records and prevent the non-prescribed payment of gamete donors for their gametes.[10] The HFEA is also obliged to maintain a code of practice which it continues to update.[11]

15.1.5 Pre-implantation genetic diagnosis (PGD) involves taking a cell from the embryo and using that cell to determine the genetic make-up of the embryo. This could simply cover the diagnosis of chromosomal or other genetic defects that might be present in the embryo. What amounts to a defect is a controversial issue. This falls into the area covered by the HFEA remit.[12]

15.1.6 A sub-category of this type of testing, sex selection, is permitted to prevent the implantation of embryos in which there is a significant risk that they may carry a serious genetic disease.[13] However, sex selection for social reasons is prohibited by the HFEA Code of Practice.[14]

15.1.7 Beyond this, genetic testing could extend to include tests that were not purely for the medical benefit of the future person that the embryo might become. The benefit may be a social benefit rather than a medical benefit (e.g. a handsome visage) or a benefit that does not fall to the person resulting from the embryo at all (e.g. the child becomes a 'saviour sibling'). It transpires that the legislative framework also places this type of morally contentious test into the sphere regulated by the HFEA.

---

7   s 3(3)(c) HFEA 1990.
8   s 41(1) *Human Fertilisation and Embryology Act 1990*.
9   Although a case cannot be brought to trial without the consent of the Director of Public Prosecutions: s 42 *Human Fertilisation and Embryology Act 1990*.
10 s 12 *Human Fertilisation and Embryology Act 1990*. The maximum a donor can receive in expenses is £50.00: Appendix G HFEA Code of Practice 2003 (sixth edition, amended).
11 s 25(1) *Human Fertilisation and Embryology Act 1990*.
12 *Quintavalle (on behalf of Comment on Reproductive Ethics) v HFEA* [2005] UKHL 28, HL.
13 paras. 14.22–3 HFEA Code of Practice 2003 (sixth edition, amended).
14 paras. 8.9 and 14.10 HFEA Code of Practice 2003 (sixth edition, amended).

15.1.8 In *Quintavalle (on behalf of Comment on Reproductive Ethics) v HFEA*[15] the legal question was not whether it was right to undertake non-therapeutic testing of an embryo (a moral issue) but whether the legal framework gave the HFEA the power to license such testing. This distinction is important because it demonstrates how Parliament has placed the value judgements[16] made in relation to this type of controversial procedure (and most likely other similarly controversial procedures in the future) into the hands of a body whose members are selected by Government.[17]

15.1.9 The other point to draw from the case is that once the 'saviour sibling' is born, the HFEA cease to have any power over whether the child can or should become a donor of regenerative or non-regenerative organs. That question falls to be decided in accordance with the legal rules surrounding tissue donation (*see* Sections 17 and 18).

Quintavalle (on behalf of Comment on Reproductive Ethics) v HFEA
[2005] UKHL 28,[18] HL

Z was a 6 year old child suffering from beta major thalassaemia. The treatment option of bone marrow transplantation was denied to him for want of a matched donor. His parents had unsuccessfully tried to conceive a child without the red cell disorder who was an HLA tissue match. Such a child would, if conceived, be able to provide HLA-matched bone marrow thereby permitting Z to receive a bone marrow transplant.

The HFEA granted a licence allowing the prenatal genetic testing to extend beyond excluding the gene defect for beta major thalassaemia, permitting also HLA testing. The basis was that the risk to the embryo associated with removing a single cell for testing would not be altered. The procedure necessitated embryo selection.

The existence of the power of the HFEA to license pre-implantation HLA tissue typing was challenged by way of judicial review (see Section 15.5.6).

Held: The HFEA could lawfully license the HLA tissue typing.

The HFEA 1990 granted the HFEA the power to license treatment services that included practices designed to determine whether embryos

---

15 [2005] UKHL 28.
16 Sheldon S, Wilkinson S. Hashmi and Whitaker: an unjustifiable and misguided distinction? *Med Law Rev.* 2004; 12(2): 137–63.
17 Schedule 1, para. 4 *HFEA 1990.*
18 *Quintavalle (on behalf of Comment on Reproductive Ethics) v HFEA* [2005] UKHL 28, para. 33.

were 'suitable' to be placed in a woman.[19] The issue of interpretation turned on whether (i) PGD alone or (ii) PGD plus HLA tissue typing were included within the word 'suitable'. Lord Brown described this word as an 'empty vessel' that required one to look to context and background in order to fill it with meaning.

The core arguments in favour of the extended meaning were:

- There was no provision in relation to sex selection within the *HFEA 1990*, implying that Parliament had intended the HFEA to be responsible for making similar decisions unimpeded by a blanket rule. In any case, Parliament had reserved power to issue regulations that could modify what treatment services could be lawfully provided under licence[20]

- Maternal preference can be a factor in determining whether an embryo can be suitable to carry. Frivolous or eugenic maternal choices fell to be regulated by the HFEA

- It would leave no gap in the statutory framework.

The difficulty with using the restricted meaning was:

- That it was difficult to draw a line between a serious gene defence and other gene defects

- There was no clear provision in the *HFEA 1990* requiring this view
- It did not appear to be the intention of Parliament to leave such technologies unregulated.

15.1.10   The HFEA guidance was initially that single cell embryo biopsy in the absence of a risk of inheriting the condition would mean that the embryo carries a risk with no clear benefit identified for the resulting child.

15.1.11   This advice was applied in the Charlie Whittaker case. Charlie Whittaker was a 3-year-old boy suffering from the sporadic condition Diamond-Blackfan anaemia (congenital pure red cell aplasia). He, too, was likely to benefit from matched-donor bone marrow transplantation.

15.1.12   Charlie's parents' request for a licence to pursue pre-implantation genetic testing to allow them to select an embryo that was HLA-matched to Charlie was refused. The Whittakers went to America and successfully conceived an HLA-matched sibling, Jamie. Charlie

---

19   ss 11(a), Schedule 2, para. 1(1)(d) and Schedule 2, para. 1(3) *HFEA 1990*.
20   Schedule 2, para. 1(1)(g) *HFEA 1990*.

received stem cell treatment using cells from Jamie in 2004.[21] The HFEA relaxed this basis for prohibition by its guidance in 2004.[22]

15.1.13 The limits of judicial intervention into the discretion of the HFEA become most clear where the clinician and the HFEA have a difference of opinion over the merits of a particular medical intervention. Whilst operating within the ambit of their lawful discretion, the HFEA are able to make decisions that can override the clinical judgements of particular clinicians.

R v The Human Fertilisation and Embryology Authority ex parte *Assisted Reproduction and Gynaecology Centre* [2002] EWCA Civ 20

H was a married 47-year-old woman. She had previously undergone eight cycles of IVF without success. Her doctor D wished to implant five embryos rather than the three which was the maximum permitted by the then-current HFEA guidance. The guidance was based on United Kingdom outcome data.

The HFEA refused to permit the use of additional embryos even after considering additional scientific data submitted by D including medical outcome data for patients treated in the USA.

H and D sought judicial review of the HFEA decision (*see* Section 15.5.6).

Held: The HFEA had acted within the bounds of their lawful discretion.

The dispute between D and the HFEA in relation to the merits of using three or five embryos turned on a conflict in the medical scientific evidence and was not one suitable to be resolved by way of judicial review.

15.1.14 The technologies continue to advance.[23] In response to a Report by the Science and Technology Committee[24] the Government has declared

---

21 http://news.bbc.co.uk/1/hi/health/3930927.stm.
22 *See* also Chico v Saviour siblings: trauma and tort law. *Med Law Rev.* 2006; **14**(2): 180–218.
23 Renwick P, Trussler J, Ostad-Saffari E, *et al.* Proof of principle and first cases using preimplantation genetic haplotyping: a paradigm shift for embryo diagnosis. *Reprod Biomed Online.* 2006; **13**(1): 110–9.
24 House of Commons Science and Technology Committee. Human Reproductive Technologies and the Law. Fifth Report of Session 2004–05 (HC-7I).

an intention to seek wider views on the question of whether regulatory intervention in the current position is merited.[25]

15.2 CONSENT

15.2.1 In addition to the HFEA, the second powerful force shaping the landscape in this area is the principle of consent. It is enshrined in Schedule 3 of the *Human Fertilisation and Embryology Act 1990*. The general legal principles of consent still operate in relation to this area of diagnosis and treatment. However, the additional statutory provisions limit what can be done with donated gametes and any resulting embryos. The general principle is that the storage and use of gametes or embryos can only be done with the consent of the donors.

15.2.2 Therefore, in the absence of consent:

(i) gametes cannot be received to be used or used for treatment purposes[26]

(ii) gametes cannot be used to create an embryo outside the body,[27] and

(iii) if created, an embryo cannot be received for treatment purposes[28] nor can it be used. (Note that this use of an embryo requires the consent from *both* the gamete donors.[29])

15.2.3 Similar principles apply to the use of embryos acquired by other means.[30] The gametes and resulting embryos can only be stored whilst the consent of the donors persist and provided the prescribed time limits have not been exceeded. The original time limits were set at five years for embryos[31,32] and 10 years for gametes.[33] These have been

---

25 Government Response to the Report from the House of Commons Science and Technology Commitee: Human Reproductive Technologies and the Law (Cm 6641) para. 44.
26 Schedule 2, para. 5 *HFEA 1990*.
27 Schedule 2, para. 6(1) *HFEA 1990*.
28 Schedule 2, para. 6(2) *HFEA 1990*.
29 Schedule 2, para. 6(3) *HFEA 1990*.
30 Schedule 2, para. 7 *HFEA 1990*.
31 s 14(4) *HFEA 1990*.
32 Schedule 2, para. 2(3) *HFEA 1990*.
33 s 14(3) *HFEA 1990*.

increased by regulation[34,35] so that storage can, in some cases such as premature infertility, continue for up to 39 years. However the age of the donor is linked to the duration of storage.

15.2.4 The basis of the principle is that the creation of children should be done with the willing cooperation of all those concerned. This operates indirectly to promote the welfare of the child. Consent as a control mechanism also provides a means to protect the autonomy of the donors in relation to the procreative choices they make.

15.2.5 The principle of consent here mirrors the principles found in the case law (*see* Chapters 3–6). Consent must be competent, voluntary and informed.[36]

15.2.6 Because of the serious and potentially contentious nature of consent in this area of law, there are formalities. The consent must be in writing and cover the purposes for which the gametes or any embryo can be used, how long these can be stored, and what is to happen to these if the person giving consent loses capacity or dies.[37]

15.2.7 Any given consent can be made subject to conditions,[38] and this consent can by varied or withdrawn by the person giving the consent until such time as the gametes or embryo have been used.[39,40] In the absence of consent and these formalities, the general principle is that storage and use of gametes and embryos is unlawful.

15.2.8 In addition to a common law duty to inform (*see* para. 6.4.8) there is a statutory obligation for the gamete donor or patient to be given the opportunity for counselling.[41,42] This counselling goes beyond general information about the processes and procedures.[43] It can include implications counselling, support counselling and therapeutic counselling.[44] This offer of counselling can be refused. However, unlike refusals to accept information in the general case law, the

---

34 *The Human Fertilisation and Embryology (Statutory Storage Period) Regulations 1991* SI 1991/1540.
35 Modified by *The Human Fertilisation and Embryology (Statutory Storage Period for Embryos) Regulations 1996* SI1996/375 – extends the potential duration of storage.
36 para. 6.3 HFEA Code of Practice 2003 (sixth edition, amended).
37 Schedule 3, paras. 1 and 2 *HFEA 1990*.
38 Sch 3 paras. 1 and 2 *HFEA* 1990.
39 Schedule 3, para. 4(2) *HFEA 1990*.
40 Schedule 3, para. 4(1) *HFEA 1990*.
41 s 13(6) *HFEA 1990*.
42 Schedule 3, para. 3(3)(1)(a) *HFEA 1990*.
43 Part 5 HFEA Code of Practice 2003 (sixth edition, amended).
44 Part 7 HFEA Code of Practice 2003 (sixth edition, amended).

fact of refusal to accept counselling can be taken into account by the treatment centre when is deciding whether to offer treatment or not.[45]

15.2.9   The net result is a framework that makes clear 'bright line' demarcations, promoting certainty and consistency in what is a controversial area of medical, legal and moral complexity. It also, cleverly, does not touch upon the question of the precise legal status of the embryo. This framework can be compared with the framework created by the *Human Tissue Act 2004* where the issue cleverly not touched upon is the question of whether human tissue amounts to property or not (*see* Chapter 18).

15.2.10 Hard cases can arise within this type of clearly demarcated and rigid framework. In the Diane Blood case, the HFEA exercised their available discretion to soften the consequences of this rule, but the precise circumstances are unlikely to recur.

R v Human Fertilisation and Embryology Authority ex parte *Blood* [1997] 2 All ER 687

P's husband died aged 30 years from meningitis. Whilst unconscious but before his death P asked the responsible doctors to collect sperm and to store it. The sperm should not have been preserved and stored in the absence of consent from the donor. However, this storage was done in good faith and in consultation with the HFEA in the context of great legal uncertainty.

P sought to use the sperm to become pregnant. However, in the absence of consent from the donor to the use of the sperm, this use, like the storage, was unlawful under the provisions of the *Human Fertilisation and Embryology Act 1990*.

The HFEA, in exercise of its discretion,[46] refused permission for the stored sperm to be exported so that treatment could be carried out abroad. This was on the basis that to permit export of the sperm would be to allow P to escape the consent provisions within the *HFEA 1990*.

P sought judicial review of this decision (*see* Section 15.5.6).

Held: The HFEA should reconsider its decision.

The HFEA had not taken two important facts into account when reaching its decision:

---

45   para. 7.3 HFEA Code of Practice 2003 (sixth edition, amended).
46   s 24(4) *HFEA 1990*.

(i) The sperm should not have been stored without the consent of the donor. This legal fact was made clear by the judgment in this case. Because it was unlawful, such storage would not be permitted in the future. The situation could not, therefore, arise again

(ii) The right of P to receive treatment in other countries under European law.[47]

The HFEA had no discretion to authorise treatment within the United Kingdom.

Post note: The HFEA did reconsider its decision and permitted Diane Blood to export her husband's sperm to Belgium. She has had two children since. She continued to successfully campaign in this area of law (see Section 15.4.9).

Practice point: In an acute situation akin to the facts of the Diane Blood case, where the parent of a couple seeking to have children is acutely ill, then if the patient is competent it is sensible to seek advice from the HFEA and consider obtaining consent to the storage and use of gametes and consequent embryos to cover the eventuality that the patient dies or becomes incompetent as a result of their illness.

15.2.11 Subsequent cases were less able to ameliorate the hard demarcations set down by the framework. A challenge attacking the validity of a withdrawal of consent was unsuccessful in the next case.

U v Centre for Reproductive Medicine [2002] EWCA Civ 565

On 6 September 2000 P's husband, who had had a previous vasectomy, gave consent for his sperm to be collected, stored and used. The sperm were surgically collected on 7 September 2000. After consultation with a specialist nurse, P's husband withdrew this consent on 25 October 2000. P's husband died suddenly and unexpectedly on 9 January 2001.

P argued that the withdrawal of consent was vitiated by undue influence.

Held: The withdrawal of consent was valid. The persuasion faced by P's husband did not overbear the independence of his decision.

---

47   Art 49/50 EC treaty.

15.2.12 A recent direct challenge to the principle of consent based on the European Convention of Human Rights was also unsuccessful. Its strongest claim was made on the basis of the right to respect for a private and family life (Article 8).

Evans v the United Kingdom [2006] ECHR 200

P underwent IVF treatment with her partner, H. P suffered borderline tumours on both ovaries requiring bilateral oophorectomy. P had eggs collected before the oophorectomy. After discussion with H and with H's consent, rather than pursue the route offered by the relatively new technology of egg freezing, a decision was made to have the eggs fertilised with H's sperm and the consequent embryos stored for further use.

After the surgery P and H separated. H subsequently withdrew his consent to allowing the embryos to be used to treat P.

P brought an action seeking to obtain access to the embryos in order that she could have a child that was genetically her own.

Held: In the absence of H's consent, the embryos could not be used to treat P.

Key arguments

For the withdrawal of consent being effective:

(i) Schedule 3, para. 6(3) of the *HFEA 1990* precludes the use of embryos without the consent of both gamete donors

(ii) P and H were no longer being treated together in the circumstances (*see* Section 15.4.5).[48]

Against the withdrawal of consent being effective:

(i) Article 2: right to life. The embryos were not legal entities within English law and so could not claim a right to life (*see* Section 12.1.12)

(ii) Article 8: right to respect for a private and family life. For P this right had been compromised, but the degree of compromise had to be balanced by the competing rights. The rights of H not to be forced to become a parent were also to be weighed under this article. P's rights under this article did not override those of H. Further, should this situation be reversed the outcome would be the same. A wide margin of appreciation was available to Nation States in this contentious area.

---

48   *Re: R (a child)* [2003] 2 All ER 131, CA.

The English legal provisions were compatible with this right. They fell within this margin of appreciation.

(iii) Claims to the right to found a family (Article 12) and the right to be free from discrimination (Article 14) only operated if the claim under Article 8 was successful.[49] A claim to a right to found a family in this case amounted to a claim to be treated with IVF. This claim did not engage the right to found a family.[50]

Against the withdrawal of consent being valid:

(i) It was argued that H had made a promise not to withdraw his consent to treatment. This promise was not established by the evidence but, even if it had been made, the *HFEA 1990* gave the right to withdraw consent (see Section 15.2.5) and this could not be overridden on policy grounds.[51]

15.2.13 Sadly, Natallie Evans did not gain access to the embryos she had created with her then fiancé Howard Johnston.

15.2.14 It is interesting to contrast this case with *Burke v GMC* (see Section 3.1.10) and *St George's NHS Trust v S* (see Section 4.5.3). In the former, consent could not be used as a sword to require treatments from medical professionals that were not medically indicated. In the latter the principle of consent formed a shield strong enough to protect the right of a mother to be free from physical interference against claims by third parties (medical staff) who sought to invade that right to protect the interests of the fetus.

15.2.15 The crucial difference in the *Evans* case was that both the parties were patients. The conflict arose between Natallie Evans's interest in having a family and private life (her procreative autonomy) and Howard Johnston's interest to choose whether he developed a family life (his procreative autonomy). In balancing these two claims to procreative autonomy, two factors appeared to be driving the decision:

(i) The requirement for mutual consent. This requirement, deriving from the *HFEA 1990*, exists in part to protect the interests of any future child

---

49 No 17142/90 Dec 10.7.91.
50 *Evans v Amicus Healthcare Ltd* [2003] EWHC 2161, Fam, paras. 261–5 per Wall J.
51 *Evans v Amicus Healthcare Ltd* [2004] EWCA Civ 727, CA para. 120 Arden LJ.

(ii) The principle of justice as symmetry. As was pointed out in the initial hearing, if the positions had been reversed, i.e. Howard Johnston became infertile and wished to use the embryos, he could not have done so without the consent of Natallie Evans.

15.2.16 Consent to licensed procedures on behalf of children cannot be given by those with parental responsibility.[52] *Gillick* competent children can consent to licensed treatment, although the extended time limits for the storage of gametes and embryos only cover children aged 16 years and above.[35,36] Gametes can only be taken from *Gillick* competent children (less than 18 years of age) if they are to treat the patient themselves or to treat the patient's partner.[53]

15.2.17 The *Mental Capacity Act 2005* explicitly excludes giving consent to licensed treatments by another person or the Court.[54]

15.2.18 From 1 April 2005 the donor of any gametes or embryos that were used during treatment under the *HFEA 1990* lost their anonymity. When a child resulting from the treatment reaches the age of 18 years they become entitled to receive specified identifying information about the donor in addition to the specified non-identifying information already available. Donors who made donations prior to the 1 April 2005 will be able to retain their anonymity.[55]

15.2.19 Conscientious objection is permitted by Section 38 of the *HFEA 1990*. It covers all activities covered by the *HFEA 1990*. It is similar to the provision found in the Abortion Act 1967 (*see* Section 14.1.12).

15.3 MATERNITY

15.3.1 The mother of the child within the terms of the *HFEA 1990* is the woman carrying the child, essentially the birth/gestational mother.[56] In the absence of techniques covered by the *HFEA 1990*, the woman carrying the child is almost certainly providing the eggs. This woman would be both the birth mother and the genetic mother. She would also be the legal mother at common law.

---

52   para. 6.11 HFEA Code of Practice 2003 (sixth edition, amended).
53   para. 3.8 HFEA Code of Practice 2003 (sixth edition, amended).
54   s 27(1)(h) *Mental Capacity Act 2005*.
55   s 31(4)(a) *HFEA 1990*; *The Human Fertilisation and Embryology Authority (Disclosure of Donor Information) Regulations 2004* SI 2004/1511. *See*, also, *Rose v Secretary of State for Health* [2002] EWHC 1593.
56   s 27 *HFEA 1990*. Transfer of an implanted embryo or of a pregnant uterus to another person are not covered or presently possible.

15.3.2 The birth mother could be genetically unrelated if the egg is placed inside the mother and fertilised by fresh sperm. This is because Section 27 of the HFEA covers the placement of embryo or sperm *and* eggs. Therefore, the placement of the egg alone may not fall within the terms of the *HFEA 1990*. It is likely, however, that if such a lacuna exists and is exposed to judicial scrutiny the Court will fill the gap in a way that harmonises the legal position.[57]

15.3.3 Other, presently fanciful, possibilities could also challenge this position. For example, if a transfer of pregnancy between women ever becomes possible then the gestational and birth mothers may be different people. No doubt these possibilities will be dealt with as they arise.

15.4 PATERNITY

15.4.1 In case law paternity is linked to genetic parentage, although there is a presumption that the husband is the father.[58] This presumption in favour of the husband as father can be rebutted by evidence that another person is the father. In modern times such rebuttal can be done powerfully by using DNA testing.[59,60]

15.4.2 Unlike the position at common law, paternity within the *HFEA 1990* is linked to social parentage. Therefore, this social element must be considered together with the consent requirements when addressing questions of paternity. Consent operates differently in relation to questions of paternity.

15.4.3 If the couple provide their own gametes then the male partner is the father. This is the case whether the couple are married or not.[61] To this extent, genetic fatherhood continues to equate to paternity.

15.4.4 If the couple are married and use donor sperm then, unless the husband does not consent to the treatment, the husband is the father. If the donor sperm is used without the husband's consent then there is no father. If the couple are unmarried and use donor sperm then the male partner is the father provided the couple are **'treated together'**.

---

57 Freeman MD. Medically assisted reproduction. In Grubb A., editor. *Principles of Medical Law*. Oxford University Press; 2004. pp. 639–738.

58 *Mater semper certa; pater est quem nuptiae demonstrant* (The mother is always certain; the father is whom the marriage shows).

59 *Leeds Teaching Hospitals NHS Trust v A* [2003] EWHC 259 (*see* Section 15.4.7).

60 *Tavli v Turkey* [2007] 1 FLR 1136 – supported by Article 8: right to a family life.

61 s 28(5) *HFEA 1990*.

15.4.5 In this last case, an unmarried couple using donor sperm, the fact that the male partner continues to consent to the treatment is not the fact that establishes paternity. In the absence of genetic parentage, the male partner's paternity is established by the fact that the couple were being treated together at the time that the gametes or embryo were placed in the woman partner.[62] Whether a couple are being treated together is a question of fact that turns on the precise circumstances of the case.[63] This imposes the obligation upon the treatment centres to keep accurate records and to reassess the situation in relation to offering treatment if the underlying relationship of the couple alters.

Re: R (a child) [2005] UKHL 33, HL[64]

P and F were unmarried. F had undergone previous bilateral orchidectomy for testicular cancer. They accepted treatment and were treated together for one cycle of treatment. At some point after this cycle of treatment their relationship broke down.

P underwent a second cycle of treatment which was successful. F never withdrew his consent to treatment.

F made an application for parental responsibility and access to the child.

Held: F was not the father either genetically, socially or legally.

At the time of the second cycle P and F were no longer together. Therefore, they were not being treated together at the time that the embryo was placed into P for the second cycle of treatment. It was no longer a joint enterprise.

15.4.6 Thus a key question, in addition to the existence of consent, is whether or not the couple being treated are pursing a shared goal together. However, the picture is not quite complete. There is a third parameter in the equation: that is the treatment actually received. Where a couple has consented to a treatment and is pursing this treatment as a joint enterprise it is possible for the treatment actually delivered to miss the area circumscribed by the consent.

---

62   s 28(3) *HFEA 1990*.
63   *Re: B (parentage)* [1996]) 2 FLR 15.
64   Also known as *Re: D (a child)* [2005] UKHL 33.

15.4.7 This occurred on the facts of *Leeds Teaching Hospitals NHS Trust v A*.[65] Here a major error made by the treatment centre created a situation that lay outside of the scope of the consent given by the couples to be treated. The result was to throw the situation outside the protections of the *HFEA 1990* and leave it to be resolved by family law principles. Thus, in a case of assisted conception, the model of social paternity embodied in the *HFEA 1990* gave way to the case law model of genetic paternity. This created both difficulties and uncertainties.

Leeds Teaching Hospitals NHS Trust v A [2003] EWHC 259, QBD

Mr A and Mrs A were a Caucasian couple who consented to IVF using Mr A's sperm and Mrs A's eggs. Mr B and Mrs B were a non-Caucasian couple who consented to IVF using Mr B's sperm and Mrs B's eggs. The treatment centre made the gross error of fertilising Mrs A's eggs with Mr B's sperm and then implanting the embryos into Mrs A. The result was the birth of healthy mixed-race twins.

The children were cared for by Mr and Mrs A. Mr and Mrs B had no contact with the children. A DNA test proved that Mr B was the genetic father. An action was brought to determine who was the legal father.

Held: Mr B was the legal father.[66]

The treatment delivered by the clinic was beyond the consent provided by both couples. No consent was given to the use of donor sperm or to the donation of sperm by either couple. Mr A and Mrs A could not be said to have been treated together[67] because the treatment they had consented to have together simply did not occur.

Mr A could not therefore take advantage of the legal machinery provided by the *HFEA 1990* to assert his paternity. On common law principles the presumption of paternity possessed by being married to Mrs A[58] was rebutted by the DNA test.[68] Therefore Mr B, the genetic father, was the legal father.

In order to become the legal father Mr A would have to adopt the twins.

15.4.8 Where the sperm or an embryo created with the sperm of a man is used after his death, then that man is not the legal father of the child.[69]

---

65 [2003] EWHC 259.
66 Article 8: right to respect for a private and family life was considered but did not impact upon the outcome.
67 Within s 28(3) *HFEA 1990*.
68 s 26 *Family Law Act 1969*.
69 s 28(6) *HFEA 1990*.

This provision was put into place in order to allow the estates of these dead men to be wound up. If they were left as potential legal fathers then the estates would have to remain administered until the legal storage period of the sperm expired or the sperm or embryos were used.[70] This could have been many years.

15.4.9 After winning her legal case, Diane Blood sought to modify this rule so that she could have the name of her deceased husband entered into the birth certificate of her children as their father. The law was changed to permit this.[71]

15.5 ACCESS TO SERVICES

15.5.1 Under Section 13(5) of the *HFEA 1990* the medical professionals responsible for providing infertility services are required to take into account the 'the welfare of any child who may be born as a result of the treatment (including the need of that child for a father), and of any other child who may be affected by the birth'.[72] The responsible medical professionals are left a degree of discretion. This leaves complex social, moral and medical issues to be resolved by a reliance on professional skills and professional integrity.

15.5.2 The HFEA Code of Practice offers guidance in this assessment. Treatment centres must have clear written criteria which set out how they make their assessment of this welfare of the child criterion.[73] The assessment must take into consideration the risk of harm to any children, including medical and social threats, as well as the couple's commitment to raise children and their ability to provide a suitable environment for any child's upbringing. The age and health of the potential parents, together with their ability to provide for the needs of the children, are also considerations.[74] The risk of harm to the patient(s) seeking treatment also impacts upon the welfare of any potential child. If there is a change in circumstances including a change of partner, a child born to the patient(s), or a long delay before treatment then the assessment must be repeated (*see* also Section 15.4.5).[75]

---

70 *Human Fertilisation and Embryology (Deceased Fathers) Act 2003* explanatory notes para. 5.
71 *Human Fertilisation and Embryology (Deceased Fathers) Act 2003*.
72 s 13(5) *HFEA 1990*.
73 para. 3.3 HFEA Code of Practice 2003 (sixth edition, amended).
74 para. 3.12 HFEA Code of Practice 2003 (sixth edition, amended).
75 para. 3.5 HFEA Code of Practice 2003 (sixth edition, amended).

15.5.3　Grounds for a refusal to offer treatment turn on the welfare of any children born as the result of the treatment, the welfare of any existing children, or a conclusion that it is inappropriate to offer such treatment.[76] Refusal can also be justified where there is insufficient available information to make a judgment.[77] If not selected for treatment then the patient(s) are entitled to know the reasons why they were not deemed suitable.[78] One such refusal to treat based on an exercise of the discretion has been unsuccessfully challenged.

R v Ethical Committee of St Mary's Hospital (Manchester) ex parte H [1988] 1 FLR 512, Fam

P sought infertility treatment. She and her husband had been refused status as potential foster/adoptive parents. P also had a history of previous convictions including loitering for prostitution.

Once the treatment centre discovered P's background she was removed from the waiting list, although P was not notified of the true basis of their decision. The clinicians had involved their hospital ethics committee in the decision-making process.

P sought judicial review (see Section 1.3.9) claiming that the decision had been made by the committee not the consultant and that P had not had the opportunity to make representations to the committee.

Held: The treatment centre had not acted unlawfully.

The committee had only given advice to the consultant on decision. P had had opportunity to make representations to the consultant and the treatment centre. There was no blanket ban fettering the discretion of the treatment centre nor had there been any procedural unfairness.

15.5.4　In considering the Human Rights aspects we have seen in *Evans v the United Kingdom*[79] (*see* Section 15.2.12) that the positive aspect of the Article 8: right to respect for a family life does not have sufficient force to fracture the requirement for consent within the terms of the HFEA 1990.

15.5.5　In the next case, the Court of Appeal refused to allow a prisoner serving a life sentence the right to use artificial insemination to found

---

76　para. 3.23 HFEA Code of Practice 2003 (sixth edition, amended).
77　para. 3.23 HFEA Code of Practice 2003 (sixth edition, amended).
78　para. 3.24 HFEA Code of Practice 2003 (sixth edition, amended).
79　[2006] ECHR 200.

a family with his wife. This was despite the claim being based on Article 8: right to a private and family life, coupled to Article 12: right to found a family.

R v Secretary of State for the Home Dept ex parte Mellor [2001] EWCA Civ 472, CA

P was in prison having been convicted of murder. P married M whilst in prison and desired to found a family. At the date of trial P was 29 years old and M was 25 years old. The earliest date that P could obtain conjugal access to M would be at the date his tariff expired. At this time P would be 34 years old and M would be 31 years old.

The medical evidence was that there was no clear evidence to suggest that M's fertility would decline sufficiently before the end of P's tariff such that artificial insemination would be medically necessary at this point in time.

P sought permission from the Secretary of State for permission to found a family by artificial insemination using fresh sperm. The Secretary of State refused permission.

P sought to challenge the decision of the Secretary of State by way of judicial review (see Section 15.5.6).

Held: The decision of the Secretary of State was lawful.

The inability to have children was social not biological. The cause for P's lawful detention was under his own responsibility.

The treatment of artificial insemination using fresh sperm was not covered by the HFEA 1990 (see para. 15.1.2).

Article 8: right to respect for a private and family life was engaged but not breached.

Article 12: right to marry and found a family. The right to found a family by conjugal means was lawfully precluded by the policy that prevented conjugal visits.[80,81] P was therefore claiming a right to found a family by artificial insemination where he was lawfully precluded from founding a family conjugally. P could not establish this right.

15.5.6   Despite this outcome, in the subsequent case of *Dickson v United Kingdom*,[82] the Grand Chamber of the European Court of Human

---

80   *X v United Kingdom* (1975) 2 DR 105.
81   *ELH and PBH v United Kingdom* (1997) 91A DR 61.
82   Application no. 44362/04 [2007].

Rights found that the Government's policy approach to this question was in breach of Article 8. In particular, there was a failure to weigh the relevant competing individual and public interests and to assess the proportionality of the restriction. Whether this reverses the policy or amends it is yet to be determined at the time of writing.

15.5.7   Where the treatment sought was publicly funded, the issues in debate surround the balance of resources available to the providing authority. In general the Court does not regard it to be its role to examine the merits of financial balancing exercises.

R v Sheffield HA, ex parte *Seale* (1995) 25 BMLR 1

P was aged 37 years and sought infertility treatment. The policy of the local Health Authority was that such treatment was only offered to people aged 35 years or less on the basis that it was more efficacious in this group. It took into account local financial constraints.

P sought judicial review (*see* para. 1.3.10 on the basis of s 3 NHS Act 1977 whereby the Secretary of State has the obligation to provide medical services that meet all reasonable needs.

Held: The decision of the Local Authority was not unlawful in light of the financial constraints.[83]

15.5.8   However the outcome might be different today. The National Institute for Clinical Excellence (NICE) has issued guidance[84] about the provision of infertility treatment services and this guidance carries a degree of legal force.[85]

---

83   Kennedy and Grubb. *Medical Law.* 3rd ed. Reed Elsevier; 2000. On page 1278 the authors point out that there may have been a case to be made for illegality on the basis of a fettering of discretion by the use of a blanket ban.
84   National Institute of Clinical Excellence. *Fertility: assessment and treatment for people with fertility problems.* 2004. http://guidance.nice.org.uk/CG11/niceguidance/pdf/English accessed 23 March 2007.
85   para. 2 and para. 4 *Directions to Primary Care Trusts and NHS Trusts in England* [2003] concerning arrangements for the funding of Technology Appraisal Guidance from the National Institute for Clinical Excellence (NICE) (www.dh.gov.uk/assetRoot/04/07/56/86/04075686.pdf) made using powers granted to the Secretary of State for Health under the *National Service Act 1977*.

15.6 CONCLUSION*

15.6.1 The basic premise is a complex statutory framework regulated by a statutory authority, the Human Fertilisation and Embryology Authority. There is great power vested in these unelected, government-appointed experts. This leads to a form of delegated expert government, an eidimocracy.

15.6.2 The legal structure uses consent as a clear demarcation to avoid having to contend with the difficult legal question of the legal and moral status of the embryo.

15.6.3 A direct comparison with the regulation of human tissue (*see* Sections 17 and 18) demonstrates how that structure also uses consent to avoid addressing the different question of the extent to which human tissue is property. The fact that both structures use the principle of consent should not lead one to be deceived into thinking that superficial similarity implies actual similarity.

---

*   This section could not include any changes that might arise from the presently proposed *Human Embryology and Fertilisation Bill 2008* (*see* para. 1.1.5).

16 Surrogacy

16.1 INTRODUCTION

16.1.1 Surrogacy is an arrangement whereby a woman agrees to become the birth mother of a child. She also agrees that after birth the child will be handed over to other persons who will then exercise parental rights over the child.[1]

16.1.2 The birth mother may or may not be genetically related to the child. For example, she may be genetically unrelated if she is treated with IVF and receives embryos created from the eggs and sperm of the putative social parents. Irrespective of this, she will always be the legal mother (*see* Section 15.3.2).

16.1.3 The determination of paternity follows the rules set out in the previous section (*see* Section 15.4). Note how the rules are modified where the circumstances of the conception fall within the terms of the *Human Fertilisation and Embryology Act (HFEA) 1990*.

16.1.4 The essential legal position is that a surrogacy arrangement is not illegal. Payments to a surrogate mother beyond her expenses are lawful.[2] This contrasts with the limits on the monies that can be paid to gamete donors and the altruism demanded from organ donors. However, such an arrangement cannot be enforced in a court of law.[3]

16.1.5 Akin to the rules on the use of human organs (*see* Section 18.10.1), the idea that third parties could make a profit from such arrangements was felt to be abhorrent. (Warnock report, Brazier Report). The consequence is that negotiating such arrangements on a commercial basis is a criminal offence.[4] Where an organisation is involved in such commercial negotiations, the organisation[5] and those in charge of

---

1   s 1 *Surrogacy Arrangements Act 1985*.
2   *Briody v St Helen's & Knowsley Area Health Authority* [2001] EWCA Civ 1010, para. 10 per Hale LJ.
3   s 1A *Surrogacy Arrangements Act 1985*.
4   s 2(1) *Surrogacy Arrangements Act 1985*.
5   s 2(5) *Surrogacy Arrangements Act 1985*.

the organisation[6] are guilty of a criminal offence. Advertisements offering or seeking surrogacy are also illegal.[7] Lack of knowledge of the existence of such activities is a good defence.[8] Non-commercial agencies, e.g. Childlessness Overcome Through Surrogacy (COTS), can exist.

16.1.6   The result of the rule that surrogacy arrangements will not be enforced is that there are risks to both sides. The putative social parents cannot be certain that they will receive the child after it is born.[9,10] Conversely, the surrogate cannot enforce promised payments, although she is in the strong position of having the child initially and of being the legal mother. If there is a dispute the Court will look to where the best interests of the child lies.[11]

16.2   CASE LAW: RIGHTS OF THE BIRTH MOTHER

16.2.1   If a surrogate mother chooses to keep the child then, in the absence of overriding issues that might affect the welfare of the child, the Court is likely to allow the child to remain with the birth mother.[12]

Re: P (minors)(wardship: surrogacy) [1987] 2 FLR 421, QBD

H and W entered a surrogacy agreement with S. The child was to be conceived by artificial insemination using H's sperm and S's eggs.

Unanticipated, S conceived identical twins. S decided that she did not wish to surrender the children. She retained custody of the children and had been with them for five months by the time of trial.

H sought custody as the genetic father. He could offer them a superior intellectual and material upbringing.

Held: Custody went to S.

The content of the surrogacy agreement did not bind the Court. S had bonded with the children.

---

6   s 2(7) *Surrogacy Arrangements Act 1985.*
7   s 3 *Surrogacy Arrangements Act 1985.*
8   s 2(9) *Surrogacy Arrangements Act 1985.*
9   *A v C* [1985] FLR 445.
10   *Re: P (minors) (wardship: surrogacy)* [1987] 2 FLR 421.
11   s 1(1) *Children Act 1989.*
12   *A v C* (1978) [1985] FLR 445.

16.2.2   If the surrogate mother chooses to surrender her rights over the child
and the parents arranging the surrogacy are suitable then the child
may go to the parents making the surrogacy arrangement.

Re: C (a minor) (wardship: surrogacy) [1985] FLR 846

The Baby Cotton case. H and W were married. W was congenitally sterile.
H and W made a commercial surrogacy arrangement with S through
an American agency. S was paid £6500. S became pregnant by artificial
insemination using H's sperm. A child (C) was born with S as the mother
and H as the genetic father. S surrendered the child.

The local authority obtained a place of safety order for the child. After an
investigation, the local authority supported H and W as parents.

Held: H and W could adopt the child.

16.2.3   It was the case that parents seeking to obtain parental rights over
a child born by surrogacy had to seek to adopt the child. This was
complex and required the Court to approve the payment made to
the surrogate mother.[13] Further, adoption meant that the surrogate
retained some rights over the child. Problems could arise where the
birth mother later sought to recover parental rights over the child.

Re: MW (adoption: surrogacy) [1995] 2 FLR 759

H and W entered a surrogacy agreement with S. The surrogacy agreement
was negotiated by the non-profit-making organisation COTS. The child was
conceived using H's sperm and S's eggs by artificial insemination. After the
birth the child was handed over to H and W. S was paid £7500.

After 2½ years S sought contact with the child, refusing her consent as
the genetic mother to an adoption order.

Held: S was unsuccessful. H and W were the parents.

The surrogacy payment was retrospectively approved by the Court. An
injunction was issued preventing S contacting the child until adulthood.

---

13   *Re: an adoption application (surrogacy)* [1987] 2 All ER 826.

16.3 STATUTE: TRANSFERRING PARENTAL RESPONSIBILITY

16.3.1 Section 30 of the *HFEA 1990* created a less arduous process when the commissioning couple are married and either one or both of them contributes gametes to the creation of the child. It permits the Court to issue an order making the commissioning parents the legal parents of the child. This can be done provided (inter alia) that the application is made within six months of the birth, the child's home is with the commissioning couple, the birth mother and her husband or the father have agreed, no payments relating to the process (other than expenses) have been made or received by the commissioning couple and at least one of the parents is domiciled in the United Kingdom.[14]

16.3.2 Because s 30(6) *HFEA 1990* bars the parental order if the consent is required of someone who cannot be found, a difficulty arose in a case where, by law, there was no father (*see* Section 15.4.4).

Re: Q (parental orders) [1996] 1 FLR 369

H and W entered a surrogacy arrangement with S who was unmarried herself. A child was conceived using IVF with the egg taken from W fertilised with donor sperm. It was a licensed treatment under the *HFEA 1990*. H and W applied for an order under Section 30 of the *HFEA 1990*. Section 30(5), *HFEA 1990* requires that the father of the child must give unconditional consent to the order.

Held: The order could be issued.

H and S were not treated together under Section 28(3) of the *HFEA 1990* and, therefore, the child had no father. (S was unmarried so s 28(2), *HFEA 1990* did not apply). Therefore, there was no legal father and so no consent from a father was required before the parental order could be issued.

16.4 CONCLUSION*

16.4.1 Surrogacy is not illegal although surrogacy for profit is illegal. Surrogacy agreements are not enforceable in law. The effect is to give the birth mother the option of parental responsibility, an option she can choose to waive.

---

14   Re: G (Surrogacy: Foreign Domicile) [2007] EWHC 2814.
*   This section could not include any changes that might arise from the presently proposed *Human Embryology and Fertilisation Bill 2008* (*see* para. 1.1.5).

17 Human tissue

17.1 INTRODUCTION

17.1.1 The specific issue in relation to the use of human tissue is: Who can do what with which tissue? Broadly the position is set out in **Figure 3** (p. 203). We can see how the *Human Tissue Act 2005* encompasses the removal, storage and use of tissue taken from deceased individuals, and the storage and use of relevant material taken from living individuals.

17.1.2 The general principle within the *Human Tissue Act 2004* is that, to remain within the law, a clear purpose must be defined for the removal, use or storage of tissue and that consent must exist in relation to that purpose.

17.1.3 For the purposes of the *Human Tissue Act 2004* human tissue includes whole bodies, organs, and pieces of tissue including DNA. However, it excludes gametes and embryos outside the body – these are governed by *Human Fertilisation and Embryology Act 1990*.

17.1.4 Part of the reason for distinguishing between a living and deceased person as the source of the tissue is that a relatively complex but effective legal structure for consent already exists in relation to living patients. Thus, removal of tissue from a living person must be justified by the consent of the individual (*see* Chapters 3–5) or have some other legal justification.

17.1.5 The *Human Tissue Act 2004* draws a distinction between complete human bodies and (relevant) tissue removed from human bodies. In **Figure 3** (p. 203), storage and use are listed under living human bodies. This is for two reasons. First to remind oneself that legal structures exist to justify both the lawful detention of living individuals and their use for medical research. And, secondly, to demonstrate how the boundary between people and human tissue (no longer a person) shapes the legal landscape.

17.1.6 The heart of the philosophical problem lies around the concept of property and its relation to the human body. We will consider this interesting idea first. We will then go on to examine the common law position before moving to examine the main provisions of the *Human Tissue Act 2004*.

Usefully the conceptual property issues and the practical consent framework are clearly separate. Therefore it is not necessary for the reader to work through the property aspects and basic common law (Sections 17.2–17.4) to make sense of the practical machinery of the consent framework provided by the *Human Tissue Act 2004* (*see* Section 18).

17.2 CONSENT AND PROPERTY RIGHTS

17.2.1 An approach based on consent as an expression of autonomy (i.e. consent as an expression of the interest in self-determination) tends to maximise the power the donor can exercise over the tissue before it has lawfully entered someone else's possession. By comparison, a proprietal right in a piece of tissue grants continuing power over the tissue even after it moves out of their possession.

17.2.2 To counter this weakness of consent the *Human Tissue Act 2004* extends the use of consent beyond an expression of autonomy by adding a role for consent as authorisation. However, even consent as authorisation does not amount to the same thing as owning something in the possession of another. (For examples *see* Sections 18.6.2–18.6.5 and 18.8.1–18.8.3).[1]

17.2.3 The importance of this distinction between using consent as authorisation and regarding donated human tissue as property is perhaps best demonstrated by the facts of the following Californian case where failure of consent was a ground of action against the physician but could not operate against an innocent third party.

---

1 *See* Herring J, Chau PL. My body, your body, our bodies. *Med Law Rev.* 2007; 15(1): 34–61.

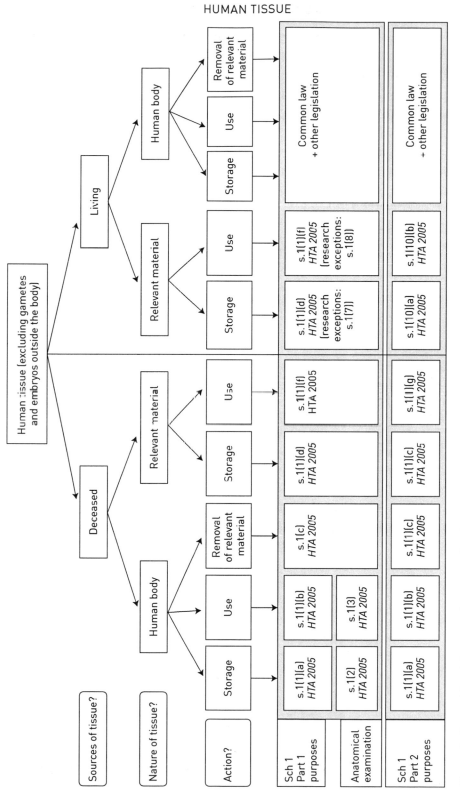

Figure 3 General legal framework surrounding human tissue. See Sections 18.1 and 18.3 for definitions.

Moore v Regents of the University of California (1990) 51 Cal.3d 120, 793 P.2d 479 Sup Ct Cal

D was responsible for P's care. P underwent splenectomy for hairy cell leukaemia. D obtained P's consent to therapeutic splenectomy but did not declare any research or financial interest in the procedure. D utilised the removed splenic cells to create a lucrative T-cell line (the Mo-cell line – used in the discovery of HTLV-2[2]). The cell line was patented by D but the rights were then passed to the Regents.

P sued D and the Regents for a share of the proceeds of the commercial exploitation on the basis that it was his cells that were the ultimate source of the profits. P made two broad claims:

(i) That the cells were taken and used without his consent[3], and

(ii) That P had a proprietary interest in the cells that should be protected.[4]

P was forced to make the latter claim because the patent was held by the Regents. They had not breached any requirement for consent. P's only claim against them was grounded in a proprietary interest in the cells.

Held (majority): P's claim against breach of consent succeeded against D. P's claim against the Regent's failed for lack of property rights vested in P.

P's consent was not fully informed because D had not disclosed the conflict of interests nor the potential uses that the tissue was to be put.

P had no property claim to the cell line because it was something new created from P's cells. P could not transform the rights protected by consent into a property right.

17.2.4 Note the subtle but important distinction between:

(i) consenting to removal and storage or use of tissue, and

(ii) the agreement to transfer property rights.

---

2   Kalyanaraman VS, Sarngadharan MG, Robert-Guroff M, *et al.* A new subtype of human T-cell leukemia virus (HTLV-II) associated with a T-cell variant of hairy cell leukemia. *Science.* 1982; **218**: 571–3.

3   The arguments surrounding the claim of breach of fiduciary duty rests in part on the conflict of interests possessed by D. Pursuing these arguments would take us into deep waters that need not be plumbed here.

4   P sued in the tort of conversion.

Transferring property rights is only possible where such rights exist in the first place. We will, therefore, move now to consider the nature of property rights, in particular how they manifest in relation to human tissue.

17.3 PROPERTY

17.3.1 The idea of property is a rich concept in law. Property is the right to utilise or dispose of something and to exclude others from interfering with that thing. One interesting and important view of the concept of property is that it is not a relationship between a person and a thing, it is a relationship between people about a thing.[5]

17.3.2 Property is more than a single right, e.g. the right of possession. It must include other rights such as the right to use the thing in certain ways. Thus ownership can be thought of as a bundle of rights.[6] Some rights can be exercised against everyone in the world[7] (e.g. owning a piece of land) others operate just against one person (e.g. someone from whom you have bought a pen).[8]

17.3.3 Property can come in distinct flavours like equitable title and ownership at law. Whilst these distinctions are not important here there is an important distinction that lies between **ownership** and **possession**. A person can possess something without owning it. Thus it is possible to have physical power over an object by possessing it yet still be bound by the rights of the owner. These concepts are generally comprehensible in relation to things like pens and land.

17.3.4 The nature of the thing that is the subject of proprietal rights is also important. Most people can readily grasp that it is possible to own tangible things like pens and land. However, the idea of property also extends to intangible things like inventions and songs or books. Rights to control inventions fall within the law of patents whilst rights to control intellectual creations such as songs or music fall within the law of copyright.

---

5   Hohfeld WN. *Fundamental legal conceptions as applied in judicial reasoning* (1919). Ashgate Publishing; 2001.

6   *See*, for example, Björkman B, Hansson SO. Bodily rights and property rights. *J Med Ethics.* 2006; **32**: 209–14.

7   Called a right *in rem*.

8   Called a right *in personam*.

17.3.5   Difficulty arises when considering the concept of property in relation to the human body. The human body lies on the boundary between a person and a thing. People can own things but not other people. (Before the end of slavery, people could own other people[9] but this is no longer true.[10]) The problem is that death is not a clear marker of the boundary between people and things. The remains of deceased people are accorded a great deal of respect in most societies. Reasons for this include respect for the dignity of the deceased person, respect for the feelings of the bereaved and other sociological reasons.

17.3.6   This societal respect prevents a human body from becoming merely a thing capable of ownership at the point of death. It is this view that prevents the body from becoming a potentially commercial object capable of being owned from the moment of death.[11] When, or indeed if, it does eventually become something that can be the subject of proprietal rights remains an open legal question.[12]

17.4   PROPRIETAL RIGHTS AND THE HUMAN BODY

17.4.1   The common law rule is that no one can own a corpse.[13,14,15,16,17,18] One consequence is that the deceased's wishes in relation to the disposal of their body after death are not enforceable at law.[19] Another consequence is that a person in possession of a corpse cannot have that possession challenged by an owner. In effect, this enlarges the rights of those who possess human tissue.

17.4.2   If someone has unlawfully come into possession of body parts, what happens if there is no owner who can claim them back? In *Doodeward v Spence*[20] the Australian High Court decided that something that cannot be property cannot be stolen. Then, by a majority, it created

---

9   *Butts v Penny* (1677) 2 Levinz. 201; *Chambers v Warkhouse* (1693) 3 Salk. 140.
10   *Smith v Gould* (1706) 2 Salk. 666; *Shanley v Harvey* (1762) 2 Eden 126.
11   Note the lessons learnt from Burke and Hare: http://en.wikipedia.org/wiki/West_Port_murders.
12   *R v Kelly* [1998] EWCA Crim 1578, [1998] 3 All ER 741, 749 per Rose LJ.
13   Blackstone W. *Commentaries on the Laws of England*. Oxford: Clarendon Press; 1765–69. Book 2, Chapter 28, p. 429.
14   *Williams v Williams* [1882] 20 Ch D 659.
15   *Doodeward v Spence* (1908) 6 CLR 406, Aust High Ct.
16   *R v Kelly* [1998] EWCA Crim 1578, [1998] 3 All ER 741.
17   *Exelby v Handyside* (1749) 2 East PC 652 (East's pleas of the Crown of 1803).
18   *A B and Others v Leeds Teaching Hospital NHS Trust* [2004] EWHC 644.
19   *Williams v Williams* [1882] 20 Ch D 659.
20   *Doodeward v Spence* (1908) 6 CLR 406, Aust High Ct.

an exception to this rule for a body that was not awaiting burial (or cremation). Armed with this exception, the Court looked to decide who had the strongest claim to possession.

Doodeward v Spence (1908) 6 CLR 406, Australian High Ct

Griffith CJ, Barton J, Higgins J

The body of a stillborn 'two-headed baby' (sic) was taken and preserved by the attending doctor in 1868. There was no evidence that consent had been obtained from the mother. Upon the death of the doctor in 1870 the preserved body was sold at auction to P's father. P subsequently acquired the body and placed it upon public display for money.

D, the sub-inspector for police, seized the body under warrant and proposed to give it a decent burial. P sought to recovery the body.

At the initial trial and upon the first appeal P's action was dismissed. P appealed again.

Held (2:1): P did have a right of action to recover the body.

Griffith CJ: There was no right of property in the dead body of a human being.[21] However, this body differed from a body awaiting burial (or cremation) in that it had been preserved for almost 40 years.

An action for possession of the body lay at the suit of a person under the duty to bury the corpse.[22] D did not have a close relationship with the child and could not demonstrate a legal duty to bury the body.

Possession of an unburied body was not itself unlawful provided it was not injurious to:

(i) public welfare

(ii) public health, or

(iii) public decency.

P had come into possession of the body in as lawful a manner as was possible.

A disturbance of lawful possession, even of a thing that could not be owned, could be remedied at law.

Barton J: Agreed with Griffith CJ. He also noted that the decision in relation to possession did not condone public display of the body.

---

21 *Exelby v Handyside* (1749) 2 East PC 652 (East's pleas of the Crown of 1803).
22 *R v Fox* (1841) 2 QBD 246 where a gaoler refused to give up possession of the body of a prisoner to executors.

Higgins J (dissent): Given there was no property in the body, then there was no reason to accept that P's claim to the body was any stronger than D's. Therefore D should be allowed to retain the body.

17.4.3 A person with a stronger claim to possess the corpse than the person in current possession can recover the corpse. For example, the executors,[23] who have a duty to bury the corpse, have a stronger right to possess the body because of this duty than someone to whom the deceased owed money.[22] In *Doodeward v Spence*[24] the police officer D could not establish that he had a duty to bury the body and so could not override P's claim to possession on this basis.[25]

17.4.4 Where the strength of claim of an executor is unclear, the power of disposal remains with the possessor of the corpse. In *University Hospital Lewisham NHS Trust v Hamuth*[26] the body was in the possession of the Hospital. The will of the deceased was in dispute. The executor under the will sought control of the body in order to arrange cremation. Other relatives sought control of the body in order to arrange burial. Given that the strength of the claim of the executor was in question, the power of disposal lay with the Hospital.

17.4.5 Note that other people may have claims on a corpse too.[25] For example, a coroner who has a duty to investigate a death[27] can claim a still stronger right to possess the corpse in certain circumstances.[28] This right is based on the State interest in preserving law and order.

17.4.6 Whatever the true position at common law, a corpse or part of a corpse falls within the definition of property within in the *Theft Act 1968*[29] if it has 'acquired different attributes by virtue of the application of skill'.[30] The effect of this is that possession or control over a body or body parts altered in such a way can amount to the statutory crime of theft.

---

23 *Re: Grandison* TLR 10 July 1989.
24 *Doodeward v Spence* (1908) 6 CLR 406, Aust High Ct.
25 *See,* also, *Dobson v North Tyneside Health Authority* [1996] 4 All ER 474, CA.
26 [2006] EWHC 1609.
27 s 8 *Coroners Act 1988.*
28 s 22 *Coroners Act 1988.*
29 s 4 *Theft Act 1968.*
30 *R v Kelly* [1998] EWCA Crim 1578, [1998] 3 All ER 741, 748 per Rose LJ.

R v Kelly [1998] EWCA Crim 1578, CA

P1 was an artist. P2 worked as a junior technician at the Royal College of Surgeons in London. P2 removed prosections (carefully and skilfully prepared anatomical specimens) for P1 to use in artistic endeavours. P1 undertook to bury the specimens after their use. P1 paid P2 £400.

Both P1 and P2 were convicted by a jury for stealing the specimens under the *Theft Act 1968.*

They appealed arguing, *inter alia*, that they could not steal something that could not be owned.

Held: The convictions were upheld.

The work done on the specimens made them something more than a corpse (or body parts) awaiting burial. This was sufficient to allow the prosections to fall into the very broad definition of property within Section 4 of the *Theft Act 1968*. As property within the terms of this Act, interference with or possession or control of the prosections could amount to theft.

The arguments that the body or body parts:

(i) might have been unlawfully held, or

(ii) were (or should have been) for burial (or cremation)

were not accepted. Note that the jury must have found that there was dishonesty on the part of P1 and P2 in order to have convicted the pair.

17.4.7   In *R v Kelly*[31] the Court built upon the decision in *Doodeward v Spence*[32] by offering a protection to the possessor of human tissue against those who might remove the tissue dishonestly. On the other side of this line is *Dobson v North Tyneside Health Authority*,[33] where making pathological slides of brain tissue in the course of a coroner's post-mortem was held to be insufficient to reduce the tissue to property.

17.4.8   What further rights might be protected remains a matter for controversy. Until the full gamut of possible rights is explored, the extent to which a human body (or body parts) can amount to property must remain uncertain.

---

31   [1998] EWCA Crim 1578.
32   *Doodeward v Spence* (1908) 6 CLR 406, Aust High Ct.
33   [1996] 4 All ER 474.

18 The Human Tissue Act 2004

18.1 GENERAL

18.1.1 The core rule is that provided the appropriate consent is obtained in relation to a lawful purpose then the removal, storage and/or use of human tissue is permitted by the *Human Tissue Act 2004*.[1]

18.1.2 We will consider a few general points then move on to consider in more detail the functions of the Human Tissue Authority before addressing the two elements of consent and statutory purposes. Return to **Figure 3** (p. 203) which sets out the essential areas covered by the *Human Tissue Act 2004*.

18.1.3 The basic structure is an ocean of liability (*see* Section 18.3.1) bridged by lawful exceptions. This has similarities to the legal structure surrounding abortion law. However, unlike abortion law, the exceptions here are more numerous and more expansive.

18.1.4 The removal of tissue from living humans is covered by the rules of consent derived from common law and other legislation (*see* Sections 3–6). The rules differ between material taken from living and deceased people (*see* Sections 18.8.1–18.8.3 and Section 18.10.6 *et seq.*). The question of whether the tissue was taken from a living person or a deceased person is judged at the point in time of the separation of the tissue.[2]

18.1.5 For the purposes of the Act the **definition of death** is to be set by the Human Tissue Authority within their codes of practice.[3] At the time of writing this definition had not yet been declared.[4] **Human body** is not defined in the Act.

18.1.6 **Relevant material** is any material consisting of or including human cells (excluding gametes and embryos outside the human body, and

---

1   s 1 *Human Tissue Act 2004.*
2   s 54(2) *Human Tissue Act 2004.*
3   s 26(2)(d) *Human Tissue Act 2004.*
4   *See* www.hta.gov.uk/_db/_documents/hta_meeting_14_february_2006.pdf paras. 11–15.

hair and nails from living individuals).[5] Embryos and gametes outside the human body are covered by the *Human Fertilisation and Embryology Act 1990* (*see* Section 15). Fetal tissue is regarded as human tissue belonging to the mother.[6]

18.1.7   Hair and nails from living people are generally excluded for pragmatic reasons, but are covered within the scope of the DNA analysis rules (*see* Section 18.11.2).

18.1.8   **Organ** is defined elsewhere as 'a differentiated and vital part of the human body, formed by different tissues, that maintains its structure, vascularisation and capacity to develop physiological functions with an important level of autonomy'.[7] The irony of even organs possessing autonomy should not be lost.

18.1.9   **Storage and use** are not defined within the Act but seem to be intended to cover all situations where human tissue might be held or utilised.

18.1.10   The functions of coroners are exempted from the *Human Tissue Act 2004*.[8,9,10]

18.2   THE HUMAN TISSUE AUTHORITY

18.2.1   We will consider here only the remit, functions and powers of the Human Tissue Authority. Broadly the **remit** covers removal, storage, use and disposal of human bodies and relevant tissue for all the purposes discussed below.[11] In addition, it also covers post-mortem examination. Post-mortem is not defined but amounts to the use of a deceased human body for the purpose of determining the cause of death. In this sense it falls into categories already present within the structure of the *Human Tissue Act 2004* (*see* **Figure 3**, p. 203 and **Table 6**, p. 214).

18.2.2   The remit of the Human Tissue Authority does not extend to blood or anything derived from blood (i.e. bone marrow or peripheral blood

---

5   s 53 *Human Tissue Act 2004*.
6   para. 66 Human Tissue Authority Code of Practice. Code 1: Consent. July 2006.
7   s 3(5) *Human Tissue Act 2004 (Ethical Approval, Exceptions from Licensing and Supply of Information about Transplants) Regulations 2006* SI 2006/1260.
8   s 11 *Human Tissue Act 2004*.
9   *See Coroner's (Amendment) Rules 2005* SI 2005/420.
10   *See* Human Tissue Authority. *Code of Practice – Post mortem examination*. Code 3 July 2006.
11   s 14 *Human Tissue Act 2004*.

stem cells) that is used in relation to transplantation,[12] except where the donor is a living incompetent adult or child (*see* Section 18.10.6). It does cover all the other tissue types set out in Section 18.1.6.

18.2.3   The Human Tissue Authority has the following **functions**:

(i)   To operate a system of licensing people and premises covering removal of tissue from the body of a deceased person, storage of human bodies or relevant material for scheduled uses (*see* **Table 6,** p. 214), anatomical examination including post mortem (which subsumes the removal of tissue),[13] and public display of deceased human bodies or relevant material removed from deceased human bodies.[14]

Human cell lines created outside of the body, including immortalised human cell lines, are not regarded as coming from a human body.[15] However, tissues and cell lines grown outside the human body and intended for human application do fall within the licensing remit of the Human Tissue Authority.[16]

(ii) To produce guidance,[17] in the form of codes of practice,[18] which must be approved by the Secretary of State.[19] These codes are not legally binding[20] but breaches of the code of practice can be taken into account when the Human Tissue Authority makes decisions in relation to licensing matters.[21]

18.2.4   It is an offence to undertake activities that need a licence without possessing one.[22] Licences are issued to designated individuals and cover people acting under the direction of the designated individual.[23,24]

---

12   s 14(5) *Human Tissue Act 2004.*
13   *See* Human Tissue Authority. *Code of Practice – Post mortem examination.* Code 3 July 2006.
14   s 16 *Human Tissue Act 2004.*
15   s 54(7) *Human Tissue Act 2004.*
16   s 7 *The Human Tissue (Quality and Safety for Human Application) Regulations 2007* SI 2007/1523.
17   s 15 *Human Tissue Act 2004.*
18   *See* www.hta.gov.uk/guidance/codes_of_practice.cfm.
19   s 29 *Human Tissue Act 2004.*
20   s 28 *Human Tissue Act 2004.*
21   s 28(2) *Human Tissue Act 2004.*
22   s 16(1) and s 25 *Human Tissue Act 2004.*
23   s 17 *Human Tissue Act 2004.*
24   The licensing requirements have exceptions in relation to tissue, for example tissue taken from living individuals, used for transplantation or research purposes: s 3 *Human Tissue Act 2004 (Ethical Approval, Exceptions from Licensing and Supply of Information about Transplants) Regulations 2006* SI 2006/1260.

18.2.5 **Powers:** The Human Tissue Authority has power to issue codes of practice; issue, revoke or vary licences (including conditional licences[25]); and hear appeals in relation to licence applications.[26] It also has the power to give directions in relation to licence holders.[27] In relation to its licensing powers, the Human Tissue Authority also has power to enter and search or inspect premises together with power to seize anything relevant to the execution of this function.[28]

18.2.6 There are also powers to dispense with consent in certain circumstances (for example, *see* Section 18.11), authorise commercial dealings in human material for transplantation purposes (*see* Section 18.10.3), and permit transplantation involving a live donor (*see* Section 18.10.9).

18.3 PURPOSES

18.3.1 Storage, use and removal of tissue are linked to purposes. It is an offence under the *Human Tissue Act 2004* to use human tissue[29] which has been consensually donated within the terms of the Act[30] for purposes other than:

(i) the Schedule 1 purposes listed in **Table 6**, (p. 214)

(ii) medical diagnosis and treatment, or

(iii) decent disposal.[31] Decent disposal includes disposal as waste.[32] Surplus tissue arising from medical diagnosis, treatment or research can be lawfully disposed of as waste, as can any tissue from a human body no longer stored to be used for a Schedule 1 purpose.[33]

18.3.2 It is also an offence to store, remove or use tissue that has been consensually donated within the terms of the *Human Tissue Act 2004* for a purpose that is not covered by the consent given.[34] When a broad consent has been obtained in relation to one lawful purpose

---

25 Schedule 3, para. 5 *Human Tissue Act 2004.*
26 Schedule 3 *Human Tissue Act 2004.*
27 Schedule 3, para. 1(5) *Human Tissue Act 2004.*
28 s 48 and Schedule 5 *Human Tissue Act 2004.*
29 'donated material' – this encompasses bodies of the deceased and relevant material from human bodies: s 8(5) *Human Tissue Act 2004.*
30 'donation' is defined in s 8(6) *Human Tissue Act 2004.*
31 s 8(4) *Human Tissue Act 2004.*
32 s 54(4) *Human Tissue Act 2004.*
33 s 44 *Human Tissue Act 2004.*
34 s 5(1)(a) *Human Tissue Act 2004.*

(*see* **Table 6**) it is possible to use the tissue for other lawful purposes provided that the consent extends to cover the other purpose or that consent is not required for the other purpose. This is particularly in relation to tissue from living donors (*see* Section 18.8.1).[35]

18.3.3   The offences are subject to a defence of reasonable belief.[36]

18.3.4   Prosecutions for use of tissue outside either the scope of the consent, or the provision in relation to which the consent was obtained, can only proceed with the consent of the Director of Public Prosecutions (DPP).[37]

TABLE 6 Purposes within the Human Tissue Act 2004.

Other purposes	Schedule 1 purposes	
	Part 1 purposes	Part 2 purposes
• Medical diagnosis and treatment. • Decent disposal. (*see* Section 18.3.1 (iii))	• Determining the cause of death. • Establishing after a person's death the efficacy of any drug or other treatment administered to him. • Transplantation. • Obtaining scientific or medical information about a living or deceased person which may be relevant to any other person (including a future person). • Research in connection with disorders or the functioning of the human body. • Anatomical examination. • Public display.	• Public health monitoring. • Education or training relating to human health. • Clinical audit. • Quality assurance. • Performance assessment.

18.3.5   The Schedule 1 purposes break down into those that involve individual patients directly (Schedule 1, Part 1 purposes), and those surrounding the mechanics of delivering a safe and effective healthcare system (Schedule 1, Part 2 purposes). The reason for this separation is to permit tissue from living donors to be used readily for Part 2 purposes whilst continuing to restrict tissue from deceased donors from being used in such ways without consent (*see* Sections 18.8.1–18.8.3).

---

35   s 5(1)(b) *Human Tissue Act 2004.*
36   For details of which *see* s 5(1) and s 8(2) *Human Tissue Act 2004.*
37   s 50(a) *Human Tissue Act 2004.*

18.3.6 The list of Schedule 1, Part 1 purposes falls into four parts:

(i) Determining the cause of death, including the effects of any treatment received during life. Obviously, this purpose cannot apply to donors who are still alive

(ii) Benefiting third parties, i.e. organ retrieval for transplantation and obtaining medical information that may be useful to third parties (e.g. genotype and phenotype)

(iii) Medical research

(iv) Anatomical examination and public display.

The list of Schedule 1, Part 2 purposes is essentially self-explanatory.

18.3.7 The Secretary of State can add to the lists of Schedule 1 purposes by regulation.[38]

18.3.8 We will focus separately on anatomical examination and transplantation (*see* Sections 18.9 and 18.10) and also consider the rules surrounding the use of DNA (*see* Section 18.11). The other purposes will be considered as they arise in this discussion.

18.4 CONSENT

18.4.1 The core rule is that provided the appropriate consent is obtained in relation to a lawful purpose then the removal, storage and/or use of human tissue is permitted by the *Human Tissue Act 2004.*[39]

18.4.2 In our discussion we will distinguish between consent as an expression of autonomy and consent as authorisation. Consent as an expression of autonomy operates to allow people to control their own lives and bodies, whilst consent as authorisation operates to control what happens to the tissue after it ceases to be part of a person.

18.4.3 A third form of consent called **deemed consent** is a form of statutory authorisation. Thus, despite the use of the term 'consent', deemed consent is neither an expression of the patient's autonomy nor of their right to authorise what is done with their tissue. Rather, it is a permission from the State to use the tissue in certain ways (*see* Sections 18.6.4–18.6.5).

38 s 8(4)(d) *Human Tissue Act 2004.*
39 s 1 *Human Tissue Act 2004.*

18.4.4 Consent as an expression of autonomy or as authorisation, given in relation to a particular purpose by a competent tissue donor, cannot be overridden by a refusal of consent by third parties (including close relatives) even after the death of the donor, provided that that consent was still operating at the time of death.

18.4.5 The existence of consent alone does not mean that the action consented to has to be carried out,[40,41] although other legal or professional obligations may require it to be carried out. This is important particularly in relation to the choices made by competent children where the views of those with parental responsibility and possibly the Court may also need to be considered.[42]

18.4.6 Consent must be competent, informed and voluntary. Consent can be withdrawn at any time (*see* Sections 4 and 5).

18.4.7 We will consider consent for anatomical examination and public display separately (*see* Section 18.9). The following points refer to consent in the context of the other purposes. The divisions within this next part of the discussion are children and adults, living and deceased donors, and competent and incompetent patients.

18.5 CHILDREN

18.5.1 A child in this context is someone less than 18 years of age.[43] The test for competence in children remains the common law *Gillick* test (*see* Section 5.3).

18.5.2 If the child is alive and competent then it is the child's consent that is required.[44] If there is conflict or doubt about the child's competence, then the views of the Court should be sought.[45] If the competent child has not made a decision in relation to consent, then a person with parental responsibility can give consent until such time as the child expresses their decision.[46] This operates to ensure that the views of a competent child are respected but fills the gap of indecision with parental responsibility. There is no scope for persons with a qualifying

---

40   *Burke v GMC* [2005] EWCA Civ 1003, CA.
41   para. 56. *Human Tissue Authority Code of Practice. Code 2: Donation of organs, tissue and cells for transplantation* July 2006.
42   para. 44 *Human Tissue Authority Code of Practice. Code 1: Consent.* July 2006.
43   s 54(1) *Human Tissue Act 2004.*
44   s 2(3) *Human Tissue Act 2004.*
45   *R v Portsmouth Hospitals NHS Trust* ex parte *Glass* [1999] EWCA Civ 1914, CA.
46   s 2(3)(c) *Human Tissue Act 2004.*

relationship (*see* Section 18.12) to make decisions in this context. When the child is alive but incompetent, the decision in relation to consent falls to a person with parental responsibility.[47]

18.5.3   If the child has died but was competent before death then a decision in relation to consent that was in force before their death continues to operate.[48] Importantly, this decision cannot be overruled by close relatives or other persons. In the absence of such a decision, including the situation where the child was incompetent, then parental responsibility again fills the gap.[49] If parental responsibility cannot fill the gap then a person in a qualifying relationship (*see* Section 18.12) can make the decision in relation to consent.[50]

18.5.4   Note how power is given to persons in a qualifying relationship only where the child is deceased. This arises because the best interests test can operate in relation to living children when a necessary exercise of parental responsibility is absent. For deceased children, any gap created by an absence of the exercise of parental responsibility is filled by the power vested in a person who is in a qualifying relationship.

18.6   LIVING ADULTS

18.6.1   Consent is required from an adult when they are alive and competent.[51]

18.6.2   For living incompetent adults, the removal of relevant material is still covered by the common law and other legislation (*see* Section 4 and also Sections 7.1.12 and 18.10.10).[52]

18.6.3   The storage and use of relevant material taken from living but incompetent adult patients is deemed to be done with consent if it is done:

(i)   either to obtain medical or scientific information that might be relevant to another person, or for the purposes of transplantation, and

---

47   s 2(3)(c) *Human Tissue Act 2004.*
48   s 2(7)(a) *Human Tissue Act 2004.*
49   s 2(7)(b)(i) *Human Tissue Act 2004.*
50   s 2(7)(b)(ii) *Human Tissue Act 2004.*
51   s 3(2) *Human Tissue Act 2004.*
52   *Re: Y (adult patient) (transplant: bone marrow)* [1996] 2 FLR 787.

(ii) by a person who believes they are acting in the best interests of the patient.[53]

Note that there is no specification for the person so acting to be medically qualified.

18.6.4 Deemed consent to storage and use of such material also operates where the purpose is a clinical trial which is authorised and conducted within the clinical trial regulations[54] or involves intrusive research which has met the requirements set out within the *Mental Capacity Act 2005*[55,56] (*see* Section 4.8.3).

18.6.5 When the loss of capacity occurs after entry into a trial, then the deemed consent operates subject to any provisions created under the powers granted to the Secretary of State by Section 34 of the *Mental Capacity Act 2005*.[57] At the time of writing, there are no such provisions, and so the common law and other legislative rules apply (*see* Sections 4.6–4.14). For such use initiated prior to the commencement of the *Mental Capacity Act 2005*, the approval by a research ethics authority is sufficient to permit deemed consent.[58]

18.7 DECEASED ADULTS

18.7.1 Where an adult has died but a competent decision in relation to consent was in operation prior to death then that decision operates.[59] It cannot be overruled by close relatives or other persons.

18.7.2 An adult does not need to formally make this decision prior to death. Instead they can appoint an adult representative who will have power in relation to this decision after their death. The appointment can be made orally in the presence of two witnesses,[60] or in writing and

---

53 s 3(2)(a) *Human Tissue Act 2004 (Persons who Lack Capacity to Consent and Transplants) Regulations 2006* SI 2006/1659.
54 *Medicines for Human Use (Clinical Trials) Regulations 2004* SI 2004/1031.
55 s 30(1)(a) and (b) *Mental Capacity Act 2005.*
56 s 3(2)(c) *Human Tissue Act 2004 (Persons who Lack Capacity to Consent and Transplants) Regulations 2006* SI 2006/1659.
57 s 3(2)(d) *Human Tissue Act 2004 (Persons who Lack Capacity to Consent and Transplants) Regulations 2006* SI 2006/1659.
58 s 3(2)(e) *Human Tissue Act 2004 (Persons who Lack Capacity to Consent and Transplants) Regulations 2006* SI 2006/1659.
59 s 3(6)(a) *Human Tissue Act 2004.*
60 s 4(4) *Human Tissue Act 2004.*

signed in the presence of one witness, or it can be incorporated into their will.[61]

18.7.3   This has analogies with lasting powers of attorney that can be created under the *Mental Capacity Act 2005* (*see* Section 4.12). However, there is one important difference: unless stated otherwise by the donor, when more than one person is appointed as a nominated representative under the *Human Tissue Act 2004*, then each representative can act independently.[62] Thus, consent from just one representative is sufficient.

18.7.4   By contrast, under the *Mental Capacity Act 2005* joint holders of lasting powers of attorney must act together unless permitted to act separately by the lasting power of attorney.

18.7.5   There is a clear shortage of human organs for transplantation.[63] The pressure to increase the supply of organs is part of the basis for this difference. The other part lies in the need for consensus surrounding difficult end-of-life decisions wherever possible.

18.7.6   The former point is underlined by the fact that if it is not reasonably practicable to contact the nominated representative for a decision within the time available to make a decision, then they can be treated as unable to give consent.[64] In such a case the appointment can be disregarded.[65]

18.7.7   If there is no decision made by the individual concerned or their nominated representative then consent can be obtained from a person in a qualifying relationship (*see* Section 18.12).[66]

18.8   LIVING AND DECEASED DONORS

18.8.1   Relevant tissue lawfully taken from living people can be stored and used without consent for all the Schedule 1, Part 2 uses listed in **Table 6**[67] (p. 214) and, if anonymised,[68] for medical research approved

---

61   s 4(5) *Human Tissue Act 2004.*
62   s 4(6) *Human Tissue Act 2004.*
63   UK Transplant. Transplant activity in the UK 2006–2007. (August 2007). www.uktransplant.org.uk/ukt/statistics/transplant_activity_report/current_activity_reports/ukt/transplant_activity_uk_2006-2007.pdf.
64   s 3(8) *Human Tissue Act 2004.*
65   s 3(7) *Human Tissue Act 2004.*
66   s 3(6)(c) *Human Tissue Act 2004.*
67   s 1(10) *Human Tissue Act 2004.*
68   para. 28 *Human Tissue Authority Code of Practice. Code 1: Consent.* July 2006.

by a research ethics authority.[69,128] Arguably these uses are subject to the common law.[70]

18.8.2   Consent for storage and use of tissue for other purposes is required. These include transplantation, obtaining information for the benefit of a third party, and for research. There is no licensing requirement for such tissue unless it is used for anatomical examination, research or transplantation purposes.[71]

18.8.3   By contrast, relevant tissue lawfully removed from a deceased person is subject to the requirement for consent even for Schedule 1, Part 2 purposes. This is to prevent a repeat of the situation that arose in Alder Hey.[72,128] The licensing requirement for such tissue is waived where it is stored for research purposes[73] or is simply being transported to be analysed for non-research purposes from licensed premises and will be returned to licensed premises after the analysis.[74]

18.9   ANATOMICAL EXAMINATION AND PUBLIC DISPLAY

18.9.1   Anatomical examination means the macroscopic dissection for anatomic purposes.[75,76] Consent for the human tissue of an individual to be stored or used for the purpose of anatomical examination or public display requires written consent of the individual signed in the presence of a witness.[77,78]

18.9.2   For an adult such consent can be incorporated into their will.[79] Note that no one else can provide consent for these purposes, not even

---

69   s 1(7),(8) *Human Tissue Act 2004*.
70   s 1(7),(8) and 5(1)(b) *Human Tissue Act 2004*.
71   Regulation 3 *Human Tissue Act 2004 (Ethical Approval, Exceptions from Licensing and Supply of Information about Transplants) Regulations 2006* SI 2006/1260.
72   Chapter 10 of the Report of the Royal Liverpool Children's Inquiry, January 2001. www. rlcinquiry.org.uk/.
73   Regulation 3(4) *Human Tissue Act 2004 (Ethical Approval, Exceptions from Licensing and Supply of Information about Transplants) Regulations 2006* SI 2006/1260 – note that ethical approval *or* pending ethical approval is sufficient in this case: Reg 3(5)(b) SI 2006/1260.
74   Regulation 3(4) *Human Tissue Act 2004 (Ethical Approval, Exceptions from Licensing and Supply of Information about Transplants) Regulations 2006* SI 2006/1260.
75   s 54(1) *Human Tissue Act 2004*.
76   For Part 2 of the HTA 2004 anatomical examination refers to human bodies: s 41(2) *Human Tissue Act 2004*.
77   s 2(6) *Human Tissue Act 2004*.
78   s 3(5) *Human Tissue Act 2004*.
79   s 3(5)(c) *Human Tissue Act 2004*.

nominated representatives.[80,81] Having obtained appropriate consent, the storage of a body for the purpose of subsequent use for anatomical examination can be done lawfully[82] once the death certificate has been issued.[83] The actual use of a human body for anatomical examination can proceed lawfully after[84] the Registrar of Births and Deaths has been notified of the death.[85,86]

18.9.3   Disposal of the body or tissue should be in accordance with the donor's wishes or, where appropriate, after consultation with the donor's family.[87]

18.10   TRANSPLANTATION

18.10.1   Commercial dealings in human material for transplantation is prohibited as a criminal offence.[88,89] The costs of transporting, storing or preparing this material do not fall within this restriction, nor do the loss of earnings suffered by the donor as a result of the donation.[90] Prosecution of this offence is subject to the consent of the Director of Public Prosecutions.[91]

18.10.2   Material that has been reduced to property by the application of human skill is excluded from the rule against commercial dealings.[92] Although it would be surprising to see anatomically prepared prosections used for transplantation, this provision can be criticised because there seems no reason why such tissue should not be restricted from being used commercially for transplantation purposes. This provision is also interesting because of its effect upon the uncertainty present in the common law concept of human tissue as property (see Section 17.4.6). The effect of this provision may be to make such material, in fact, legally capable of being property.

---

80   s 2(5)(b) and s 12 *Human Tissue Act 2004.*
81   paras. 46, 49, 61 *Human Tissue Authority Code of Practice. Code 1: Consent.* July 2006.
82   s 1(2) *Human Tissue Act 2004.*
83   Under s 22(1) *Births and Deaths Registration Act 1953.*
84   s 1(3) *Human Tissue Act 2004.*
85   In accordance with s 15 *Births and Deaths Registration Act 1953.*
86   para. 24 *Human Tissue Authority Code of Practice: Code 4: Anatomical examination.* July 2006.
87   para. 28 *Human Tissue Authority Code of Practice: Code 4: Anatomical examination.* July 2006.
88   s 32 *Human Tissue Act 2004.*
89   For xenotransplantation *see* McLean S, Williamson L. The demise of UKXIRA and the regulation of solid-organ xenotransplantation in the UK. *J Med Ethics.* 2007; **33**(7): 373–5.
90   s 32(7) *Human Tissue Act 2004.*
91   s 50(a) *Human Tissue Act 2004.*
92   s 32(9)(c) *Human Tissue Act 2004.*

18.10.3 Of concern is the power granted to the Human Tissue Authority to permit commercial dealings in human material for transplantation.[93] The effect of this provision is to make immune from prosecution anyone who the Human Tissue Authority designates as someone who can lawfully pursue commercial dealings.

18.10.4 Although this provision is curtailed in relation to living donors (because the Human Tissue Authority must ensure that no reward has been received in exchange for such donations, *see* Sections 18.10.8–18.10.9), this power can still be criticised on the basis that its breadth is unnecessarily wide. For example, it potentially allows the Human Tissue Authority to sanction a market in cadaveric organs.[94,95]

18.10.5 The use of **cadaveric material** for transplantation is subject to the rules of consent discussed above (*see* Sections 18.4–18.6). Storage of tissue for the purposes of transplantation, whether the tissue comes from a living or deceased donor, is free from any licensing requirement provided that the tissue is stored for less than 48 hours. It can be stored for longer than this if the tissue is an organ or part of an organ that will replace the function of a full organ system in the recipient.[96]

18.10.6 Special rules exist in relation to **living donors** (both adults and children) to cover the removal of organs[97] or parts of organs for the purposes of transplantation. When the donor is an incompetent child or incompetent adult, this cover also extends to bone marrow and peripheral blood stem cells.[98]

18.10.7 In addition, there is a restriction best imagined as a lake of illegality bridged by a single exception that is overseen by the Human Tissue Authority. The Human Tissue Authority ensures that there is no organ trafficking, and that consent or a common law justification is present before donation and transplantation can proceed.

---

93   s 32(3) *Human Tissue Act 2004.*
94   Anand KP, Kashyap A, *et al.* Thinking the unthinkable: selling kidneys. *BMJ.* 2006; **333**(7559): 149.
95   Truog, RD. The ethics of organ donation by living donors. *NEJM.* 2005: **353**(5): 444–6.
96   Regulation 3(3) *Human Tissue Act 2004 (Ethical Approval, Exceptions from Licensing and Supply of Information about Transplants) Regulations 2006* SI 2006/1260.
97   Organ is defined in s 3(5) *Human Tissue Act 2004 (Ethical Approval, Exceptions from Licensing and Supply of Information about Transplants) Regulations 2006* SI 2006/1260. *See, also,* s 9 *Human Tissue Act 2004 (Persons who Lack Capacity to Consent and Transplants) Regulations 2006* SI 2006/1659 for a list of organs.
98   Human Tissue Authority. *Code of Practice. Code 6: Donation of allogeneic bone marrow and peripheral blood stem cells for transplantation.* July 2006.

18.10.8 The mechanics of this restriction lie in the creation of two offences in relation to the type of transplantable tissue[99] described. These offences are knowing removal and knowing use of the transplantable tissue for the purpose of transplantation. Once again, these are subject to a defence of reasonable belief,[100] where a person can establish that they reasonably believed that they were acting within the exception. Prosecution of both these offences is subject to the consent of the Director of Public Prosecutions.[101]

18.10.9 These offences can be avoided where:

    (i) the clinician responsible for the care of the donor has involved the Human Tissue Authority in the case

    (ii) the Human Tissue Authority is satisfied that there is no reward for the donor in exchange for the donation, and

    (iii) consent has been given by the donor; or that the donation is otherwise lawful.[102] These last five words,[103] in effect, import through a back door the common law rules of consent, thus permitting them to operate in relation to the removal of organs from living patients for the purpose of transplantation.

18.10.10 Consent is required from competent adults. However, in relation to incompetent adults or any child, it is deemed by the Human Tissue Authority to be good practice that the decision to proceed with removal of tissue for the purposes of transplantation should be sanctioned by the Court.[104] For children, good practice also requires that those with parental responsibility should be consulted.[105]

18.10.11 The Human Tissue Authority is obliged to take particular care in cases where the living donor is a child or an incompetent adult and the donated tissue is replacing the full function of a single organ system in

---

99 'transplantable tissue' is widely defined in s 10 *Human Tissue Act 2004 (Persons who Lack Capacity to Consent and Transplants) Regulations 2006* SI 2006/1659. It is not transplantable tissue if it is removed primarily for the treatment of the donor: s 10(2) SI 2006/1659.

100 s 33(5) *Human Tissue Act 2004*.

101 s 50(a) *Human Tissue Act 2004*.

102 s 11(2),(3) *Human Tissue Act 2004 (Persons who Lack Capacity to Consent and Transplants) Regulations 2006* SI 2006/1659.

103 s 11(3)(b)(ii) *Human Tissue Act 2004 (Persons who Lack Capacity to Consent and Transplants) Regulations 2006* SI 2006/1659.

104 paras. 22, 28 Human Tissue Authority Code of Practice. *Code 2: Donation of organs, tissue and cells for transplantation.* July 2006.

105 para. 33 Human Tissue Authority Code of Practice. *Code 2: Donation of organs, tissue and cells for transplantation.* July 2006.

the recipient.[106] It should also take particular care where the donor is a living competent adult but the recipient is neither genetically related nor known to the donor. Specifically, the Human Tissue Authority must take special steps before permitting paired donations, pooled donations and non-directed altruistic donations.[107]

18.10.12 **Paired donation** is essentially when donor1 knows or is genetically related to recipient1 and donor2 knows or is genetically related to recipient2 but, for compatibility reasons, the donations proceed as donor1→recipient2 and donor2→recipient1. This cross-linking can be increased beyond two pairs, thus amounting to **pooled donations**.

18.10.13 **Directed donation** is donation to a recipient who is genetically or emotionally related to the donor.[108] Directed donation by a competent adult can be approved more readily by the Human Tissue Authority using reports prepared by local independent assessors.[108]

18.10.14 **Non-directed altruistic donation** is something else entirely. This is where a donor offers their organ to an unknown, non-genetically-related individual (e.g. whosoever is compatible and highest on the waiting list) for purely altruistic reasons. This is an interesting ethical topic in its own right.[109]

18.10.15 **Domino transplants** arise where removal of the donated tissue is for therapeutic purposes for the donor (who receives a transplant from another source) and some or all of the tissue removed can be used for transplant purposes in the recipient. These can be considered as a series of single transplants where there is no cross linking akin to paired or pooled donations. Because there is generally a living donor, the Human Tissue Authority must be involved in order to receive the benefit of the exception described above (*see* Sections 18.10.8–18.10.9). Where the donation is directed this can be relatively straight forward.

18.10.16 In cases of non-directed domino donation the Human Tissue Authority guidance does not regard Human Tissue Authority approval as being

---

106 s 12 *Human Tissue Act 2004 (Persons who Lack Capacity to Consent and Transplants) Regulations 2006* SI 2006/1659.
107 s 12(4),(5) *Human Tissue Act 2004 (Persons who Lack Capacity to Consent and Transplants) Regulations 2006* SI 2006/1659.
108 para. 93 *Human Tissue Authority Code of Practice. Code 2: Donation of organs, tissue and cells for transplantation.* July 2006.
109 Roff SR. Self-interest, self-abnegation and self-esteem: towards a new moral economy of non-directed kidney donation. *J Med Ethics.* 2007; **33**: 437–41.

necessary.[110] This can be argued to be incorrect because in order for the Human Tissue Authority to discharge its duty it must be satisfied, inter alia, that the donor did not receive any reward for the donation and also that consent was obtained for both therapeutic removal of the donated organ and the subsequent use of the organ for transplant purposes. Whatever the position, anyone following the Human Tissue Authority guidance would be entitled to claim the defence of reasonable belief.

18.10.17 If part of a body that is lying in a hospital or other institution is suitable for transplantation, then retention of the body and the minimum necessary and least invasive steps for preserving the transplantable parts are permitted.[111,112]

18.10.18 No licence is required for storing human tissue for the purposes of transplantation provided the tissue is held for less than 48 hours. It can be held longer without a license if it is an organ (or part organ) that will replace the complete functioning of an organ system in the recipient. This is true irrespective of whether the tissue is cadaveric or from a living donor.[113]

18.10.19 Information about transplant operations[114] must be passed to an authorised body;[115] currently this is the NHS Blood and Transplant.[116,117] Interestingly, skin grafts (excluding face transplants), corneas and heart valves are not covered by this regulation.[118]

110 para. 103 *Human Tissue Authority Code of Practice. Code 2: Donation of organs, tissue and cells for transplantation.* July 2006.
111 s 43 *Human Tissue Act 2004.*
112 *See,* also, British Transplant Society. *Guidelines relating to solid organ transplants from non-heart beating donors.* Triangle Three Ltd; 2004.
113 Regulation 3(3) *Human Tissue Act 2004 (Ethical Approval, Exceptions from Licensing and Supply of Information about Transplants) Regulations 2006* SI 2006/1260.
114 ss 4, 5 and Schedules 1 and 2 *Human Tissue Act 2004 (Ethical Approval, Exceptions from Licensing and Supply of Information about Transplants) Regulations 2006* SI 2006/1260.
115 s 34 *Human Tissue Act 2004.*
116 s 5 *Human Tissue Act 2004 (Ethical Approval, Exceptions from Licensing and Supply of Information about Transplants) Regulations 2006* SI 2006/1260.
117 A Special Health Authority created by the *NHS Blood and Transplant (Gwaed a Thrawsblaniadau'r GIG) (Establishment and Constitution) Order 2005* SI 2005/2529. www. uktransplant.org.uk.
118 Regulation 9 *Human Tissue Act 2004 (Persons who Lack Capacity to Consent and Transplants) Regulations 2006* SI 2006/1659.

18.11 DNA

18.11.1 The general rules constraining the removal, storage and use of tissue also apply to DNA. The added twist is that possession of DNA with the intention to analyse it without consent for a purpose that is not permitted within the *Human Tissue Act 2004* is an offence.[119] Fortunately there are a number of exceptions.

18.11.2 The offence covers human DNA in material taken from a human body, including hair, nails and gametes; it excludes embryos outside the body.[120] However, if the material does not come from a human or does not contain human cells, then it is not covered.[121]

18.11.3 To avoid committing an offence, consent to analysis of the DNA is required plus the analysis must be for a purpose permitted by the Act (*see* Sections 18.11.9).[122]

18.11.4 The rules for <u>consent</u> to use DNA mirror those for consent set out above except that there is no provision for nominated representatives.[123] In the absence of consent, a number of exceptions exist through which the DNA analysis can be justified.

18.11.5 The consent of an **incompetent adult** is not obtainable. However, DNA can be analysed without consent where:

(i) this is believed to promote the best interests of an incompetent adult, or

(ii) the analysis is for the purposes of research (*see* Section 18.11.8 (iv)).[133]

18.11.6 An **incompetent child** requires consent to be given on their behalf by someone with parental responsibility. There is no specific provision to permit DNA analysis in the best interests of an incompetent living child in the situation where no person with parental responsibility can be found.

18.11.7 For a **deceased child**, any decision in relation to consent in force at the time of death trumps the decision of someone with parental responsibility which in turn trumps the consent of someone in a

---

119 s 45(1) *Human Tissue Act 2004.*
120 s 45(2) *Human Tissue Act 2004.*
121 s 45(5) *Human Tissue Act 2004.*
122 s 45(1)(a)(i) *Human Tissue Act 2004.*
123 Schedule 4, para. 2 *Human Tissue Act 2004.*

qualifying relationship. This is the same for a deceased adult, except that there is no one with parental responsibility.

18.11.8 **Exceptions:** On practicable grounds exceptions to the need for consent exist where:

(i) the tissue was already held prior to 1 September 2006 (when this provision came into force[124]) and the person whose DNA it is cannot be identified nor is likely to become identified, or

(ii) the tissue is very old, and where the source is a person who died both before 1 September 2006 and 100 years before the date of analysis.[125]

18.11.9 **DNA analysis is permitted** for a large number of purposes. These include:

(i) For the purpose of medical diagnosis or treatment of the person who is the source of the DNA.[126]

(ii) Where the tissue comes from a living person:

   a) for the Schedule 1, Part 2 purposes listed in **Table 6**[127] (p. 214) (i.e. those purposes supporting delivery of the health-care system), and

   b) for the purpose of medical research approved by a research ethics authority[128] where the samples are adequately anonymised.[129]

(iii) For competent living adults, for the purpose of analysing their DNA to obtain information that might benefit another person. This purpose can be authorised by the Human Tissue Authority[130] where there is no refusal of consent in place and:

   a) the competent donor cannot be found and there is no reason to believe that the donor has died or is incompetent,[131] or

---

124 s 3(2) *Human Tissue Act 2004* (Commencement No. 5 and Transitional Provisions) Order 2006. SI 2006/1997.
125 s 45(2) *Human Tissue Act 2004.*
126 Schedule 4, para. 5(1) *Human Tissue Act 2004.*
127 Schedule 4, para. 8 *Human Tissue Act 2004.*
128 s 2 *Human Tissue Act 2004 (Ethical Approval, Exceptions from Licensing and Supply of Information about Transplants) Regulations 2006* SI 2006/1260.
129 Schedule 4, para. 10 *Human Tissue Act 2004.*
130 For more details see the HTA guidance: www.hta.gov.uk/guidance/non-consensual_dna_analysis.cfm.
131 Schedule 4, para. 9(2) *Human Tissue Act 2004.*

b) if found, the competent donor cannot or has not made a decision about consent despite notice that a decision is required.[132]

(iv) For incompetent adults, for the purpose of analysing their DNA if it is believed to be in their best interest, or for a fully approved clinical trial (including intrusive research where the terms of the *Mental Capacity Act 2005* are complied with, *see* Section 18.6.4).[133] For both these permitted purposes, consent is not required from the incompetent adult.

(v) For the purpose of enabling the functioning of the legal justice system including coroners, courts and the police, and for the purposes of national security.[126]

(vi) And where the tissue was held prior to 1 September 2006, for all the purposes listed in **Table 6**, (p. 214) except anatomical examination and public display.[134]

18.12 QUALIFYING RELATIONSHIPS

18.12.1 The *Human Tissue Act 2004* provides a hierarchical ranking of close relationships (*see* **Table 7**) with people in the same rank being treated equally.[135] The method is to seek consent from the person of the highest available rank.[136] If two people are equal in the hierarchy then consent from either one will suffice.[137] A person in the hierarchy can be excluded if they do not wish to deal with the question, they are unable to deal with the question or it is not reasonably practical to communicate with them in the available time (*see* also Section 18.7.6).[138]

---

132 Schedule 4, para. 9(3) *Human Tissue Act 2004.*
133 s 5 *Human Tissue Act 2004 (Persons who Lack Capacity to Consent and Transplants) Regulations 2006* SI 2006/1659.
134 Schedule 4, para. 7 *Human Tissue Act 2004.*
135 s 27(5) *Human Tissue Act 2004.*
136 s 27(6) *Human Tissue Act 2004.*
137 s 27(7) *Human Tissue Act 2004.*
138 s 27(8) *Human Tissue Act 2004.*

TABLE 7 Ordered list of qualifying relationships within the *Human Tissue Act 2004*.[139,140]

Spouse, civil partner[141] or partner
Parent or child
Brother or sister
Grandparent or grandchild
Child of a brother or sister
Stepfather or stepmother
Half-brother or half-sister
Friend of longstanding

18.12.2 This ranking mechanism should not be used when there are serious disagreements between family members in relation to transplantation and when the benefits of donation might be outweighed by the resulting harm caused.[142]

18.13 CONCLUSION

18.13.1 This framework has resonance with the consent framework created by the *Human Fertilisation and Embryology Act 1990* which, in turn, is overseen by the Human Fertilisation and Embryology Authority (*see* Section 15.1.1). One consequence of this resonance is that proposals are in train that are likely to result in the combination of these organisations into a single body called the Regulatory Authority for Tissue and Embryos (RATE), as well as an overhaul of the *Human Fertilisation and Embryology Act 1990*[143] (*see*, also, Section 15.6.1).

18.13.2 The difficulty is that the superficial harmony between these two frameworks reflects a similar solution to different sensitive issues. For reproduction, these include the values to be placed upon fetal life and reproductive rights. For human tissue, the key issue is the precise scope of any property interest in human tissue. These questions are masked but not completely removed by the consent-based framework in the *Human Tissue Act 2004* (*see* Sections 17.2.1–17.2.3).

---

139 s 27(4) *Human Tissue Act 2004*.

140 s 54(9) *Human Tissue Act 2004*.

141 *Civil Partnership Act 2004 (Overseas Relationships and Consequential, etc. Amendments) Order 2005* SI 2005/3129 Schedule 4, para. 12.

142 paras. 55 and 57 *Human Tissue Authority Code of Practice. Code 2: Donation of organs, tissue and cells for transplantation*. July 2006.

143 www.hta.gov.uk/about_hta/how_we_work/rate.cfm.

19 End of life

19.1 INTRODUCTION

19.1.1 A number of complex principles come into play when a possible outcome is the death of the patient. The aim of this discussion is to consider the legal framework for this situation from the perspective of the medical professional. To begin to unravel and expose these complex principles, *see* **Figure 4** (below).

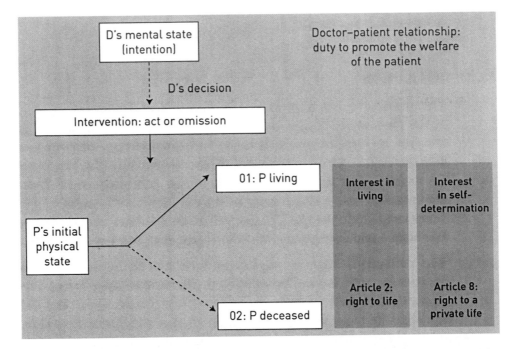

Figure 4 The Medical Factual Matrix: Overview of the various elements that should be considered in cases involving end-of-life decisions. The patient (P) begins in an initial state that, over time, moves towards an outcome state where either P remains alive (outcome 1 = O1) or dies (outcome 2 = O2). We can mark the actual course of events with a solid line. Thus, in the example given in this figure P remains alive but, clearly, we can redraw this as appropriate to any particular set of facts. P has several interests that impact upon this matrix. The medical professional's (D's) mental state incorporates elements including what D foresees, intends and desires. The D-P relationship is widely pervasive, surrounding and penetrating the entire structure. The nature of the proposed medical intervention is also important.

19.2 THE MEDICAL DUTY OF CARE

19.2.1 From **Figure 4** we can see that D's decision is made in the context of a medical professional–patient relationship which imports a duty of care owed by D to P. This imposes a duty upon the medical professional to promote the welfare of their patient. This medical duty of care is widely pervasive in extent, but there are limits to its scope. For example, a responsible medical professional has a duty of care to a patient suffering from persistent vegetative state but the scope of that duty does not extend to delivering artificial hydration and nutrition where that would be futile.

19.2.2 This duty of care owed by D to P is another route by which P's interests influence D's decision in relation to the proposed intervention. For example, P's claim to respect for their autonomy is particularly powerful when made to D because D's respect for P's autonomy is a powerful way for D to promote P's welfare.

19.2.3 The best interests of the patient influence the decision made by D in more than one way. They are an important factor in determining the scope of the duty of care for incompetent patients (*see* Section 4.7 and Section 5), and they can also operate as a justification for invading the interest in personal physical integrity when coupled with the doctrine of necessity (*see* Sections 4.7.3 and 19.8).

19.2.4 Thus for incompetent patients, determination of what are the patient's best interests lies at the heart of the treatment decision. This is particularly so where a lack of competence to consent to the proposed treatment and the question of the extent of appropriate care co-exist. This is demonstrated in the next case where an application was made, inter alia, to declare lawful both:

    a) the insertion of a percutaneous endoscopic gastrostomy tube (PEG), and

    b) the omission to provide cardiopulmonary resuscitation (CPR) in the event of cardiopulmonary arrest (a DNAR order).

Re: R (adult: medical treatment) [1996] 2 FLR 99, Fam

Sir Stephen Brown P

    P was a frail (5 stone), incompetent adult man who suffered multiple problems including cerebral palsy, epilepsy, severe constipation, recurrent lower respiratory tract infections and oesophageal ulceration.

The medical evidence was that P had little real cognitive awareness but could interpret events in his environment. It was felt that a DNAR order could be justified on grounds that CPR would be unlikely to succeed should cardiopulmonary arrest occur.

P remained for active treatment but a DNAR order including the mother's signature was issued. The day-care centre staff queried whether the DNAR order was lawful.

The Trust sought inter alia a declaration that it was lawful to insert a PEG and to issue a DNAR order.

Held: Both the DNAR order and PEG insertion were lawful.

19.3   THE INTERESTS POSSESSED BY P

19.3.1   P has certain interests that carry weight in the process of medical decision-making. These can impact upon the medical decision-making process through the duty of care that D owes to P (*see* Section 19.2.1). Alternatively they can operate through a claim to human rights or to natural rights. **Figure 4** (p. 230) identifies three key interests grounded in the *Human Rights Act 1998*.

(i)   There is the interest in living. This can influence the decision made by the medical professional through a need to have respect for the sanctity of human life. The claim for this respect is based on the view that human life has intrinsic value, a value that some argue is irreducible.[1]

An interest in living can influence the medical decision through a claim for a right to life based on Article 2 of the *Human Rights Act 1998*. The interest in life possessed by the patient cuts to the heart of the obligation owed by the medical professional to their patient because all the goods of life are contingent on the possession of life. However, whilst there is a strong presumption in favour of life-saving treatment, this presumption is not irrebuttable.

(ii)   There is the interest in self-determination, an interest that P has in being able to determine the course of their own life. This interest in self-determination is the basis of P's claim that the medical professional should act in a way that respects P's personal autonomy.

---

1   Keown J. Restoring moral and intellectual shape to the law after *Bland*. LQR. 1997; **113**: 481.

This interest can also influence the medical professional's decision through arguments based on Article 8 of the *Human Rights Act 1998*, the right to a private and family life. Article 8 also imports the interest in being free from unlawful physical interference.[2] In English law this interest is protected by the tort of battery which has been developed to provide increased protection for the principle of personal autonomy through the law of consent (*see* Section 3.3).

(iii)   There is a right to be free from inhuman and degrading treatment arising from Article 3 of the *Human Rights Act 1998*. This claim might arise when P is suffering the terminal stages of a debilitating illness and seeks to receive only palliative care or even euthanasia from D.

19.4   THE INTERACTION BETWEEN THE DUTY OF CARE AND THE INTERESTS POSSESSED BY P

19.4.1   The duty of care owed by a medical professional is to promote the welfare of the patient not to merely preserve their life. In almost all cases the preservation of life will be integral to promoting the welfare of the patient. However, as *Bland* demonstrates, there are situations where mere existence can be regarded as insufficient to impose duties upon third parties, even in situations where there is a medical professional–patient relationship in existence.

19.4.2   A medical professional is not bound to provide a treatment merely because it is demanded by a competent patient. When a competently demanded treatment is not 'clinically indicated' there is no duty to provide such treatment. However, when the treatment is 'clinically indicated' (*see* Section 3.1.10) it is a breach of duty not to provide it in the absence of a justification.[3] The provision of a non-clinically indicated life-shortening treatment can amount to a culpable homicide (*see* Section 19.6) or the crime of assisting suicide[4] when they cannot be justified either in terms of the doctrine of double effect or the acts and omissions doctrine, or by some other basis.

19.4.3   When a patient competently refuses life-saving treatment the medical professional is obliged not to undertake such treatment unless they

---

2   *R v Portsmouth Hospital NHS Trust* ex parte *Glass* [1999] EWCA Civ 1914.
3   *Burke v GMC* [2005] EWCA Civ 1003.
4   s 2(1) *Suicide Act 1961*.

can invoke some other legal justification for invading the patient's right to be free from unjustified physical interference (*see* Section 3.1). Notice that this protection for patient autonomy rests on the interest the patient has in protecting themselves from unjustified physical interference. In English law this right of competent refusal to offered medical treatment does not rest upon an interest in dying. The recognition of an interest in dying would damage the principle of sanctity of life that is so highly prized by the law.

19.4.4　The euthanasia debate is, in part, about the idea that it is morally right that the law should recognise a claim based upon an interest in dying. The assertion that no claim that rests upon an interest in dying can be made in English law was challenged in the next case when a competent patient made a competent demand to be killed. P was unsuccessful in the English Courts, so sought to challenge the decision in the European Court of Human Rights.

19.4.5　The Article 2 right to life creates a negative obligation upon the state requiring it to refrain from intentional and unlawful killing.[5] It also imposes a positive obligation upon the state requiring it to take steps to preserve the lives of those people within its jurisdiction.[6] It does not confer a power upon individuals to impose upon others the obligation to act to end one's own life. In essence, it does not create a claim right[7] to die based upon an interest in dying.[8]

Pretty v United Kingdom [2002] ECHR 423

P was a 43-year-old woman who suffered motor neurone disease. She had progressed rapidly from diagnosis three years earlier to a state of general paralysis from the neck down. Her speech was impaired from motor weakness and she required naso-gastric feeding. She was likely to die from respiratory failure in a period of weeks to months.

P sought to end her life but required the assistance of her husband. Assisted suicide is a crime in the United Kingdom under Section 2(1) of the *Suicide Act 1961*. By *Section 2(4)* of the *Suicide Act 1961* the approval of

---

5　*Osman v United Kingdom* (1998) 29 EHRR 245.
6　*Keenan v United Kingdom* (2001) 33 EHRR 38.
7　Hohfeld WN. In: Cook WW, editors. *Fundamental Legal Conceptions as Applied in Judicial Reasoning.* New Haven, CT: Yale University Press; 1919 (reprint 1964).
8　For another perspective *see* Freeman M. Denying death its dominion: thoughts on the Dianne Pretty case. *Med Law Rev.* 2002; 10(3): 245–70.

the Director of Public Prosecutions (DPP) is required for any prosecution brought under Section 2(1) of the Act.

P sought an undertaking from the DPP that he would not consent to the prosecution of her husband should the husband assist P's death. The DPP refused to provide this undertaking.

P sought judicial review of this decision and ultimately lost her case in the House of Lords.

She appealed to the European Court of Human Rights inter alia that her right to life under Article 2 of the European Convention on Human rights had been breached.

Held: P's right to life had not been breached. Article 2 did not confer a right to die.

The State had not caused P's predicament. P received medical care sufficient to meet her medical needs. P's Article 3 right to be free from inhuman and degrading treatment had to be in harmony with her Article 2 right to life and was not breached.

19.4.6   In the converse situation there is an advance competent request for life-preserving treatment to be delivered after the patient becomes incompetent. Here such a request cannot bind medical practitioners where the best interests of the patient, once incompetent, do not support continuing the life-preserving treatment.[9] This is because the scope of the duty owed by the medical professional to an incompetent patient only extends to provide treatment that can promote the welfare of the incompetent patient. Where the treatment cannot promote the welfare of the patient, an advance competent patient request for this treatment, which is to be delivered after the patient becomes incompetent, lacks sufficient force to impose a professional obligation on the medical professional to act (*see*, also, Section 3.1.11). There is no professional duty to act. In this naked situation the basic reality is simply that of one person asking another to do their bidding. A gloss on this result is the fact that the medical professional is obliged by their duty of care not to cause detriment to P by their actions or omissions (*see* also Section 19.9).

---

9   *Burke v GMC* [2005] EWCA Civ 1003.

19.5 ACTS AND OMISSIONS

19.5.1 The nature of the intervention in **Figure 4** (p. 230) can arguably be characterised as either an act or an omission. The doctrine of acts and omissions operates in relation to this characterisation of the intervention. This doctrine has regard to the actual actions undertaken or not undertaken and how they impact upon the trajectory of events.

19.5.2 The difficulty with the acts and omissions doctrine is that it can lead to such philosophical contortions that many argue that the distinction between acts and omissions is indefensible.[10]

19.5.3 For example, consider a ventilator-dependent patient on a ventilator. A timer switches off the ventilator every 12 hours and must be reset to continue ventilation. Is failing to reset the timer an omission given removing the plug from the socket is an action? The questions are:

(i) Is there actually any difference between the two situations?

(ii) And, if so, is this difference morally relevant?

19.5.4 Despite its philosophical shortcomings, the acts/ omissions distinction remains embedded in the case law.

19.5.5 Another example of this questionable distinction concerns the difference between withholding and withdrawing treatment. This variant of the acts/omissions distinction looks at how the intervention is altered rather than the nature of the intervention itself. It has been held not to have legal significance.[11] It is philosophically unclear why this should lack legal force whilst the distinction between acts and omissions does have legal force.

19.5.6 There is an important interaction between the acts and omissions doctrine and the duty of care that a medical professional owes their patient. There is no criminal liability[12] or civil liability[13] for omissions to act[14,15] unless there is a duty of care which requires action.[16] The existence of a duty of care will make an omission of care culpable where the act of delivering the care would have promoted the welfare of the patient.[15,16]

---

10 *See* especially *Airedale NHS Trust v Bland* [1992] UKHL 5, [1993] 1 All ER 821, 885 per Ld Mustill.

11 *Airedale NHS Trust v Bland* [1992] UKHL 5, [1993] 1 All ER 821, 879–880 per Lowry Ld.

12 *R v Gibbins* (1918) 13 Cr App R 134.

13 *Bolitho v City & Hackney HA* [1997] UKHL 46, HL.

14 *R v Instan* [1893] 1 QB 450.

15 *Airedale NHS Trust v Bland* [1992] UKHL 5, [1993] 1 All ER 821, HL.

16 *R v Stone* [1977] 2 All ER 341.

19.5.7 The combination of the doctrine of acts and omissions with negation of the duty of care by the principle of value futility formed the basis of the decision in the famous PVS case of *Airedale NHS Trust v Bland*[15] which is discussed below (*see* Section 19.10.1).

19.6 HOMICIDE, INTENTION AND THE DOCTRINE OF DOUBLE EFFECT

19.6.1 **Homicide:** Murder and manslaughter are criminal offences that operate to uphold and protect the sanctity of human life within society. Murder is where a person unlawfully causes the death of another with the intention of causing death or very serious bodily harm.[17,18] This includes the shortening of a life. Manslaughter is where there is unlawful killing, with a culpable mental state that does not amount to intention to cause death or very serious bodily harm, or where there is a partial defence to a charge of murder such as diminished responsibility, provocation or action in pursuit of a suicide pact.

19.6.2 **Intention** is a matter that falls to the jury to decide in the context of homicide.[17] It differs from motive or desire. It should be inferred from all facts.[19] Important facts that permit the existence of intention to be inferred include that death or serious injury was:

(i) a virtually certain consequence of the intervention[20]

(ii) foreseen as a certain or virtually certain consequence of the intervention, or

(iii) the aim of the intervention.

19.6.3 Foreseeing (or, indeed, desiring) that the intervention will shorten life, by itself is not sufficient to make the intervention culpable as murder. The death or grievous bodily harm must be an *intended* consequence of the intervention.[17,18]

19.6.4 When an intervention undertaken by a medical practitioner causes or hastens the death of a patient, then the **doctrine of double effect** may be triggered. If the medical practitioner undertakes the intervention intending to cause the outcome of death then they are culpable for homicide. On the other hand, if the medical practitioner foresees the

---

17   *R v Moloney* [1985] 1 All ER 1025, HL.
18   *R v Hancock and Shankland* [1986] 1 All ER 641, HL.
19   *R v Woollin* [1998] 4 All ER 103, Crim CA.
20   s 8 *Criminal Justice Act 1967* precludes discovering intent solely on the basis of the natural and probable consequences of the intervention.

death but intends an outcome that benefits the patient then they are acting lawfully.

19.6.5   The key is that the same intervention must cause both the beneficial outcome and hasten death. It is this coupling of good and evil flowing from the same act that forces us to look at the state of mind of the agent as the means of attributing praise or blame for the action (*see*, also, Section 19.8.5). Note that the legal question is about the culpability of the person making the decision to act.[21]

19.6.6   By operation of the doctrine of double effect, it is not murder when:

(i)   a medical practitioner in pursuit of their duty of care undertakes an intervention intended to promote the welfare of their patient, and

(ii)   an incidence of that intervention is the shortening of the life of the patient.

R v Bodkin Adams [1957] Crim LR 365, Central Criminal Court

P was a widow who had suffered a stroke and had severe arthritis. D was P's general practitioner. D had prescribed P large doses of morphine and diamorphine in addition to other drugs. P subsequently died.

   D was charged with murder. At the time of this case, murder carried the death penalty.[22]

Jury verdict: D acquitted.

19.6.7   During summing up in *Bodkin Adams* [1957][23] Justice (later Lord) Devlin stated:

> 'If the first purpose of the medicine – the restoration of health – can no longer be achieved, there is still much for the doctor to do, and he is entitled to do all that is proper and necessary to relieve the pain and suffering even if measures he takes may incidentally shorten life.'[24]

---

21   Williams G. The principle of double effect and terminal sedation. *Med Law Rev* 2001; 9(1): 41–53.

22   The death penalty was later abolished by the *Murder (Abolition of the Death Penalty) Act 1965*.

23   *R v Bodkin Adams* [1957] Crim LR 365, Central Criminal Court.

24   *See*, also, *R v Carr* Sunday Times Nov 1986; *R v Lodwig* TLR 16 Mar 1990; *R v Moor* [1999] Crim LR 2000.

19.6.8   On the other side of this line is the following case.

R v Cox (1992) 12 BMLR 38, Winchester Crown Court

Lillian Boyes (P) was a 70-year-old lady who suffered chronic illness. She was apparently terminally ill and suffering from severe pain. D (a rheumatologist) injected her with potassium chloride at her request thereby killing her.

D was charged with attempted murder rather than murder because the body had been cremated making it impossible to prove that the potassium chloride had been the cause of death.

The medical evidence was that there was no other way left to relieve her pain. The issue was whether D intended to kill P.

Jury verdict: D was convicted of attempted murder. D was sentenced to one year's imprisonment, suspended for 12 months.

19.6.9   Here the potassium chloride had no therapeutic or analgesic effects. The fact that P had requested death did not prevent the conviction. The consent of the victim is not a defence to a charge of murder where death was caused by a positive act.[25,26,27,28]

19.7   THE RELATIONSHIP BETWEEN ACTS/ OMISSIONS AND THE DOCTRINE OF DOUBLE EFFECT

19.7.1   The doctrine of acts and omissions looks to the physical character of the intervention whilst the doctrine of double effect looks to the intention of the person undertaking the intervention (*see* **Table 8**, p. 240 and **Figure 4**, p. 230). Note how intention is not part of the doctrine of acts and omissions. Note, also, that the presence or absence of the duty of care impacts upon whether culpability is imposed in cases of omission.

---

25   *R v Coney* (1882) 8 QBD 549 per Stephen J.
26   *R v Brown* [1993] 2 All ER 75, HL.
27   *R v Arthur* (1981) 12 BMLR 1 per Farquharson J.
28   *Airedale NHS Trust v Bland* [1992] UKHL 5, 39 per Mustill Ld.

TABLE 8 Criminal culpability for homicide and its relations to both the acts/omissions doctrine and the doctrine of double effect.

	Act	Omission
Intend to cause death	Murder/culpable homicide.	Not culpable homicide unless duty of care obliges action to preserve life.
	R v Cox	*Airedale NHS Trust v Bland*
	(Section 19.6.8)	(Section 19.10.1)
Not intend to cause death	Not murder if doctrine of double effect operates.	Only culpable homicide (but not murder) if the duty of care obliges action and this duty is breached recklessly or by gross negligence.
	R v Bodkin Adams	*R v Adomako*[29]
	(Section 19.6.4)	(para. 8.2.1)

19.7.2   Thus, to reach a conclusion in a particular case we must consider the intention of the agent, the nature of the intervention they have undertaken and, in the case of an omission, understand whether they have a duty to act to preserve the life or not.

19.7.3   In *Re: B (a minor) (wardship: medical treatment)*[30] (*see* Section 19.12.3) the Court determined that the surgeon's duty lay in favour of undertaking bowel surgery in a child with Down's syndrome. For the surgeon this precluded the option of omitting to undertake surgery, a course which was preferred by the parents. Contrast that case with the next case.

R v Arthur (1981) 12 BMLR 1, Leicester CC

P was a baby suffering Down's syndrome. D wrote in the notes: 'Parents do not wish it to survive, nursing care only.' D prescribed high doses of dihydrocodeine (5 mg q 4h). The baby died.

P was charged with attempted murder.

The question for the jury was whether D had acted to palliate the situation or whether D had sought to bring about the death of the child.[31]

Jury verdict: D acquitted.

---

29   [1994] 3 All ER 79.

30   *Re: B (a minor) (wardship: medical treatment)* (1981) [1990] 3 All ER 927.

31   Smith & Hogan in *Criminal law* (6th ed.) Butterworths p. 52 felt the better view is that this failure should be equated with an act causing death.

19.7.4 In *R v Arthur*[32] presumably the jury accepted that the opiates were to relieve any suffering rather than to cause death. Given the result of the case, the duty of care that D owed to the baby must be presumed not to have obliged treatment for the baby.

19.7.5 Both cases arose from a doctor–patient relationship involving a patient suffering Down's syndrome. Yet in *Re: B (a minor) (wardship: medical treatment)*[33] there was a duty to treat that precluded an omission to operate, whilst in *R v Arthur*[34] the case turned on whether the act of giving the opiates was intended to cause death.

19.7.6 From this pair of cases we can see that the basic medical facts are important but they do not determine the legal analysis. The nature of the intervention and the intention of the person undertaking the intervention are critically important.

19.8 THE PRINCIPLE OF NECESSITY AND THE CASE OF THE SIAMESE TWINS

19.8.1 This model was powerfully explored by the unusual and particular facts of the Siamese twins case.[35] Here surgical separation of conjoined twins was permitted by the Court despite the fact that it was foreseen and inevitable that one of the twins would die as a result of the positive act of surgery. The case was one of justified action causing death.

Re: A (children) (conjoined twins: surgical separation) [2000] EWCA Civ 254, [2000] 4 All ER 961, CA

Brooke, Robert Walker and Ward LJJ

J and M were one-month-old ischiopagus (joined at the ischium), tetrapus (having four lower limbs) conjoined twins. There were cloacal abnormalities including a shared bladder and separate imperforate ani. Apart from the bladder, there were no other shared organs.

J's neurological status was assessed as normal. M had reduced cortical development, partial agenesis of the corpus callosum and a Dandy-Walker malformation. There was uncertainty to the extent that M suffered pain. She was likely to suffer delayed development.

---

32 (1981) 12 BMLR 1.
33 [1981] 1 WLR 1421.
34 (1981) 12 BMLR 1.
35 *See* also Hewson B. Killing off Mary: was the Court of Appeal right? *Med Law Rev* 2001; 9(3): 281–98.

M's heart was dilated with poor ventricular function and resultant poor cardiac output providing only about 10% of her perfusion requirement. J supported M's cardiac output through a shared aorta with venous blood returning to J via a united inferior vena cava. The oxygenated blood provided to M by J's circulation was also important because M had severe pulmonary hypoplasia.

The medical evidence was that M could not survive independently in light of these cardio-respiratory abnormalities.

The available options were:

(i) Permanent union – The medical evidence was that this option would almost inevitably result in J suffering high-output heart failure over time. In this event, it was likely that both twins would die. Survival of the conjoint twins to more than six months was estimated to be only 10–20%, but with wide confidence limits.

(ii) Surgical separation:
   a) This would inevitably invade M's bodily integrity and lead to M's death
   b) There was no medical benefit in undergoing the surgery from M's perspective
   c) Urgent separation in the event of acute deterioration was estimated to carry 60% risk of mortality for J. Elective separation was estimated to carry only a 6% risk for J
   d) Surgical separation with coupled cardiac transplantation for M was not a realistic option.

J and M's parents were strict Roman Catholics from the Maltese island of Gozo. They opposed surgical separation predominantly in light of their religious views.

Held: Could lawfully undertake elective separation.

The probability was that M would die first. Should that event occur there was a high risk to J from emergent separation. Therefore, elective separation was preferable.

19.8.2   The facts left an exquisitely finely balanced set of interests.[36] The Court determined that J and M were distinct individuals, each protected by the law of murder. Therefore, the doctors owed a separate legal duty of care to each twin. The *Human Rights Act 1998* was not yet in force

---

36   *See* also *Queensland v Nolan* [2001] QSC 174.

but none of the judges felt that it would alter the decision. Despite the precise wording of the provisions in the *Human Rights Act 1998* the same rights were held both by J and by M.

19.8.3 In relation to the law of intention for murder, the Court concluded that, after the decision in *R v Woollin*,[19] the doctors did have sufficient intention for the crime of murder. In *Woollin* a father had thrown his three-month-old son onto a hard surface causing a skull fracture and subsequent death. The father had not desired the death of his son and denied any intention to kill the child. Despite this, the jury found he had sufficient intention and convicted him of murder. The conviction was reduced to manslaughter on appeal because of a misdirection to the jury at the initial hearing.

19.8.4 This view of the doctors' intention was reached despite the existence of non-binding judicial views[37] expressed in previous cases to the effect that a doctor acting in good faith in the discharge of their duty of care could not possess a guilty mind in respect to *bona fide* medical treatment.[38] In essence, the Court found that the medical nature of the procedure did not distinguish the Siamese twins case from *Woollin*.

19.8.5 The escape route of using the doctrine of double effect as a justification for undertaking the operation was also closed.[39] This was because the intention to save J could not justify the breach of duty involved in killing M. The benefit fell to J but the harm upon M. Thus apparent limits are placed upon the doctrine of double effect. These are that:

(i) the benefit and harm flowing from the act must fall on the same individual, and

(ii) no duty of care should be breached by the act.

19.8.6 The acts and omissions doctrine could not be used to justify the operation because there was a duty to act to preserve both the life of M and of J. Thus, an omission to supply J's blood to M by clamping the connection between the two aortae would still be culpable as a breach of duty.

19.8.7 At first instance Johnson J and, on appeal, Robert Walker LJ were both drawn to a view based on *Bland*. They concluded that the best interests

---

37   *obiter dicta.*

38   *Gillick v West Norfolk and Wisbech Area Health Authority* [1985] 3 All ER 402 at 413 per Ld Fraser of Tullybelton and at 424 per Ld Scarman.

39   For a counterview *see* Uniacke S. Was Mary's death murder? *Med Law Rev.* 2001; 9(3): 208–20.

of M lay in favour of the operation or at least not against surgery. Thus, the duty not to operate disappeared permitting this type of omission. However, with respect to these views, it is submitted that the better view is the view of the majority of the Court of Appeal. Their view was that purely from M's perspective it was not in her best interests to shorten her life by any surgical procedure.

19.8.8   This left the doctors with a tragic choice: by operating they would breach their duty to M, whose best interests lay in not having the operation, but by not operating they would breach their duty to J, whose best interests lay in elective surgical separation.

19.8.9   The Court was bound to act on the principle that the child's welfare is paramount.[40] This principle operates most powerfully where the competing interests do not belong to other children. When the countervailing interest is the welfare of another child, the two interests have to be balanced against each other.[41]

19.8.10   Given the balance of interests in this case, the Court concluded that elective surgery was the 'lesser of two evils'.[42] This was the key value judgement made in the case. It rested on the view that M was pre-designated to die.[43] Despite protestations that the judgment was not based on a utilitarian calculus[44] and that due regard was not being paid to the intrinsic value of M's life, it is hard to escape the brutal utilitarian logic that most could be saved from a tragic situation by elective surgery.

19.8.11   Having reached this essentially moral judgment, the fact remained that the operation would shorten the life of M and amount to the crime of murder unless a legal justification could be found.[45] To justify the surgery the Court turned to consider the legal doctrine of necessity. Necessity is the legal justification used when discharging the duty to treat incompetent adults in their best interests. It justifies the invasion of the incompetent adult's right to be free from unjustified physical

---

40   s 1 *Children Act 1989*.
41   *Birmingham City Council v H (a minor)* [1994] 1 All ER 12.
42   *Re: A (children) (conjoined twins: surgical separation)* [2000] 4 All ER 961, 1015 per Ward LJ.
43   The concept of pre-designation for death has been heartily and rightly challenged by John Harris (*see* footnote 51).
44   *Re: A (children) (conjoined twins: surgical separation)* [2000] 4 All ER 961, at 1014, 1048, 1065 approving Wilson J in *Perka v R* [1984] 13 DLR (4th) 1; at 1037–8, 1049 noting how necessity is a utilitarian doctrine.
45   Note how M's life could have been terminated lawfully had abortion been undertaken prior to birth.

interference.[46] Here the problem was that it had to operate to justify the invasion of M's interest in continuing to live.

19.8.12 In *R v Dudley and Stephens*[47] three sailors were convicted of the murder of a cabin boy, Richard Parker. During a storm the sailors and cabin boy had been cast away from the yacht *Mignonette* in an open lifeboat, 1600 miles away from the Cape of Good Hope. After 19 days at sea with limited food and water, in order to survive they killed the weakened boy Richard Parker and fed upon his body until they were rescued four days later. The sailors were found guilty of murder despite a plea of necessity.[48]

19.8.13 The principle of that case was that the powerful interest that Richard Parker had in living could not be invaded on the basis that the three sailors had decided that it was necessary to kill him in order to preserve their own lives.[49] Thus, whilst the law permits an innocent to kill an assailant (a wrongdoer) in self-defence of his own innocent life, it does not permit the killing of an innocent in order to preserve another innocent life, even if that innocent life is your own.[50,48]

19.8.14 To escape this reasoning, Ward LJ considered a form of quasi-self defence that might operate against an innocent threat. On this view, M was an innocent threat to J's life and the doctors could justify their operation on the basis that the removal of an innocent threat to J's life was lawful. This argument lacks the force to select between surgery or non-surgery because it works equally against both J and M.[51] However, it might operate as a justification for surgery once a conclusion on the value judgement in the case has been reached. Invoking this justification avoids the need to use the defence of necessity.

19.8.15 Returning to the necessity argument, the deep reason for the conclusion in *R v Dudley and Stephens*[52] is that people should not be allowed to breach legal principles on the basis that they believe it is justified in pursuit of some higher value. The problem with widening the defence of necessity lies in allowing individuals to decide what is necessary in their own interests.

---

46 *F v West Berkshire Health Authority* [1989] 2 All ER 545.
47 *R v Dudley and Stephens* [1884] 14 QBD 273.
48 Their death sentence was subsequently commuted to six months' imprisonment.
49 *Perka v R* [1984] 13 DLR (4th) 1.
50 Hale's Pleas of the Crown, vol. i: 51.
51 Harris J. Human beings, persons and conjoined twins: an ethical analysis of the judgment in *Re: A. Med Law Rev.* 2001; 9(3): 221–36.
52 (1884) 14 QBD 273.

19.8.16 In *Re: A (children) (conjoined twins: surgical separation)*[53] Brooke LJ addressed the problem head on. He looked to the deep reason for the decision in *R v Dudley and Stephens*[54] and concluded that in *Re: A (children) (conjoined twins: surgical separation)*[55] the danger of widening the scope of the defence to accommodate the surgical separation was small. He did not feel that, in this case, the defence would divorce the law from morality.

19.8.17 In order for the defence of necessity to operate, the action had to:

(i) avoid 'inevitable and irreparable evil'

(ii) be 'no more than is reasonably necessary for the purpose to be achieved', and

(iii) inflict evil only proportionate to the evil avoided.[56]

In the rare and particular facts of *Re: A (children) (conjoined twins: surgical separation)*,[57] given the tragic choice faced by the doctors (*see* para. 19.8.8), the defence of necessity could operate in relation to any charge of murder. On this basis, the elective surgical separation was approved by the majority of the Court of Appeal.

19.8.18 Comment: On balance, it appears that the basis of the pivotal moral judgment was utilitarian.[58] The most attractive legal explanation is the use of the defence of necessity, but this still begs a number of questions.

19.8.19 The 20-hour elective separation procedure was undertaken at St Mary's Hospital in Manchester when the twins were three months old. J survived; sadly, M did not.

19.9 MEDICAL FUTILITY

19.9.1 There is no duty to treat a patient where that treatment is futile.[59]

'... for my part I cannot see that medical treatment is appropriate or requisite simply to prolong a patient's life when such treatment has no therapeutic

---

53 [2000] 4 All ER 961.
54 (1884) 14 QBD 273.
55 [2000] 4 All ER 961.
56 *Re: A (children) (conjoined twins: surgical separation)* [2000] 4 All ER 961, 1050.
57 [2000] 4 All ER 961.
58 McEwan J. Murder by design: the 'feel-good factor' and the criminal law. *Med Law Rev.* 2001; 9(3): 246–58.
59 *Re: L (A Minor)* [2004] EWHC 2713, Fam, para. 12 per Butler-Sloss P.

purpose of any kind, as where it is futile because the patient is unconscious and there is no prospect of any improvement in his condition.' – Per Ld Goff in *Airedale NHS Trust v Bland* [1993], HL.[60]

19.9.2 The problem is determining when a particular treatment is futile. Looking back at **Figure 4** (p. 230) we find that at the heart of the problem is a choice faced by a medical professional (D's decision) in relation to the care of their patient. The medical professional (D) has a choice to undertake or not to undertake some intervention that can alter the likelihood of P reaching O1 or O2. Futility can arise in one of ways:

(i) The intervention cannot alter the likelihood of P reaching O1 or O2. We can call this **goal futility** because the goal of making a difference cannot be achieved.

(ii) The intervention can alter the likelihood of reaching O1 or O2 but the value of changing this likelihood is zero. Unlike goal futility, in this case we must reach an assessment of the value of the goals we are trying to achieve. We can therefore call this **value futility**.

19.9.3 Note that there is a difference between something that has no benefit (i.e. is futile) and something that might confer either benefit or harm but, after careful assessment, is judged not to be in the best interests of the patient.[61]

19.9.4 *Re: C (a minor) (medical treatment)*[62] (*see* Section 19.12.9) is an example of goal futility. The *Bland* case (*see* Section 19.10.1) is an example of value futility. In both cases, the goal can be regarded as preservation of life. In *Re: C (a minor) (medical treatment)* [1998] the intervention was artificial ventilation, whilst in *Bland* the intervention was the provision of artificial hydration and nutrition. In *Re: A (children) (conjoined twins: surgical separation)*[63] (*see* Section 19.8.1) medical futility did not operate unless one accepted that M's continuing existence was without value to her.

19.9.5 The relationship between futility and the duty of care is interesting. If we regard futility as the point where there is no benefit from the treatment then the duty of care effectively disappears. The magnitude

---

60 *Airedale NHS Trust v Bland* [1993] 1 All ER 821, 870 per Ld Goff.
61 *Airedale NHS Trust v Bland* [1993] 1 All ER 821, 868 per Ld Goff.
62 [1998] 1 FLR 384, Fam.
63 [2000] 4 All ER 961.

of the obligation imposed by the duty of care does not become positive or negative; it becomes zero. This distinguishes it from a position where there is a benefit from the treatment (positive duty to treat) or where harm results from the treatment (positive duty not to treat). In a futile situation, it can be argued that there is simply no duty of care at all.

19.9.6   The point is that if there is no duty of care in situations of futility, then it can be argued that the decision in such cases should not be made by reference to the duty of care. Thus, an additional logical step taken by the Court is to use the standard of care (i.e. the *Bolam* test as modified by *Bolitho* – *see* Section 10.4) as a yardstick of how far to go in cases of futility.

19.10   PERSISTENT VEGETATIVE STATE

19.10.1   The facts of the Tony Bland case[64] required that the House of Lords examine closely the duty of care and how it interacted with the various other principles active in the situation. It is a case that repays study.

Airedale NHS Trust v Bland [1992] UKHL 5, [1993] 1 All ER 821, HL

Keith Ld, Goff Ld, Lowry Ld, Browne-Wilkinson Ld and Mustill Ld

Tony Bland (P) was a 21-year-old man who had suffered hypoxic brain damage secondary to a severe crushed-chest injury sustained during the Hillsborough football disaster in Liverpool on 15 April 1989. By 1992, he had been diagnosed as suffering from persistent vegetative state. P was insensate and had no hope of recovery. He was dependent upon artificial hydration and nutrition (ANH), including naso-gastric feeding, for his continuing survival.

The consensus of medical opinion was that ANH should be withdrawn. The family agreed with this view.

The specific issue was whether or not it was lawful to withdraw the ANH, thereby causing his death.

It was argued that the doctors in the case owed P a duty of care as their patient. This duty was to promote the welfare of P. P's welfare included the continuance of his life, and this depended upon the doctors continuing to provide ANH. Because the duty of care required the provision of ANH it should continue to be provided irrespective of whether the intervention was an act or an omission. To withdraw ANH with the intention of causing the death of P in such circumstances would *prima facie* amount to murder.[64]

Held: Withdrawing ANH was lawful.

It would be unlawful to positively kill P. However, a failure to provide ANH was an 'omission to struggle' not a positive act akin to the act of killing in *R v Cox* (*see* Section 19.6.8).[65] There was no distinction between withholding and withdrawing ANH.[11,66]

To assess the existence and scope of the duty of care, attention had to be paid to what interests of P might be served by continuing ANH. By virtue of his existence, P did have an interest in life; however this interest, like the principle of the sanctity of life, was not absolute. For example, it would give way to a right of self-determination[67] and in cases of self-defence.[68] P did not have an interest in dying.

ANH was part of the medical treatment delivered to P.[69] It involved an invasion of P's bodily integrity[70] and, as such, it had to be justified. The purpose of medical treatment was to benefit the patient.[71] The scope of the duty of care owed by medical professionals to their incompetent patients was determined by the test of best interests (*see* Section 7). The test of best interests (at the time) was the *Bolam* standard *simpliciter*.[72]

By the principle of futility the duty of care does not extend to situations where the purpose of medical treatment cannot be achieved.[67,73] Given P's irretrievable insentience, his interest in living had disappeared.[74] ANH merely prolonged an insentient life with no hope of recovery. It was not possible to make any meaningful comparison from P's perspective about the value to P of the difference between an insensate existence versus death.[75]

The Court agreed with the medical opinion that continuing ANH was (value) futile on the facts and thus not in the best interests of P. Thus, the duty of care did not require the provision of ANH.

---

64 [1993] 1 All ER 821, 879–880 per Ld Browne-Wilkinson.
65 [1993] 1 All ER 821, 866–7 per Ld Goff.
66 [1993] 1 All ER 821, 874 per Ld Lowry.
67 Per Keith Ld [1993] 1 All ER 821, 860.
68 Per Ld Goff [1993] 1 All ER 821, 865.
69 [1993] 1 All ER 821, 870 per Ld Goff.
70 [1993] 1 All ER 821, 882 per Ld Browne-Wilkinson.
71 [1993] 1 All ER 821, 859 per Ld Keith.
72 *F v West Berkshire Health Authority* [1989] 2 All ER 545.
73 *Auckland Area Health Board v Attorney General* [1993] 1 NZLR 235, NZ High Court – withdrawal of care permitted from a patient suffering Guillain-Barré syndrome complicated by severe CNS damage.
74 [1993] 1 All ER 821, 893 per Ld Mustill.
75 [1993] 1 All ER 821, 859–60 per Ld Keith.

Because failing to provide ANH was an omission, if there was no duty to provide ANH then it would be lawful to withdraw ANH, even if one possessed the intention that it would cause P's death.12,16 Civil liability would be precluded in the absence of a breach of the duty of care.[76]

In reaching this conclusion, account was taken of the burden of the treatment including its invasiveness, the indignity to P and the distress to his family.

19.10.2   The doctrine of double effect could not operate in *Bland* because there was no mixture of benefit and harm flowing from the single intervention of withdrawing ANH. The conclusion was that P had no interest in dying. Further, it appeared that there was sufficient foreseeability and factual causal connection between withdrawing the ANH and P's death that a jury may have fairly inferred an intention to cause death.

19.10.3   This is the key point about the case. The law permits a doctor to intentionally cause the death of a patient where the duty of care is extinguished and the death results from an omission of treatment. However, if the duty of care is not extinguished, then the death of the patient in such a situation can amount to both a civil wrong and the crime of murder (*see* **Table 8,** p. 240).

19.10.4   This conclusion has been interpreted to accord with the State's obligation under the European Convention of Human Rights.

NHS Trust A v M; NHS Trust B v H [2001] 1 All ER 801, Fam

Butler-Sloss P

M and H were both women in clearly diagnosed persistent vegetative state, and were being cared for in different hospitals. M was 49 years old and had suffered peri-operative hypoxic brain injury abroad. H was 36 years old with a history of pancreatitis. She had suffered hypoxic brain injury during asystolic cardiac arrest. H was not clinically stable.

The families supported the applications to be allowed to withdraw ANH, but an organisation called ALERT opposed the application.

Held: ANH could be withdrawn in both cases.

---

76   *Airedale NHS Trust v Bland* [1993] 1 All ER 821, 883 per Ld Browne-Wilkinson.

A person with PVS is alive because the brain stem remains intact. Thus the Article 2 right to life was considered.[77,78]

The withdrawal of ANH was intended to bring about the death of the patient. The obligation to preserve life under Article 2 is not absolute. An omission to provide life-sustaining treatment informed by the best interests of the patient and made in accordance with a respectable and responsible body of medical opinion would discharge the State obligation under Article 2.

The Article 3 right to be free from inhuman or degrading treatment is not breached. It is not degrading because withdrawal of ANH is not designed to arouse feelings of fear, anguish and inferiority in the patients.[79] Generally, objectively, therapeutically necessary treatment is not inhumane or degrading.[80] Palliative treatment and respect for the patient's dignity would continue until death.

The Article 8 right to a private life protects personal autonomy (see Section 5.5.5) and is not breached in this case.

19.10.5 Current Court guidance requires that all cases of withdrawal of ANH in PVS patients should be considered by the Court before treatment is withdrawn.[81] This is to permit a body of case law to develop surrounding these difficult issues.[82] In this context if a decision is made to continue care then the religious beliefs of the patient prior to the illness should not be disregarded when planning future care.[83]

19.10.6 Withdrawal of ANH without Court involvement can amount to serious professional misconduct.[84]

---

77 *Widmer v Switzerland* App No 20527/92 (10 February 1993, unreported) – failure to make passive euthanasia illegal was not in breach of the European Convention of Human Rights.
78 A confusion arises within this judgment as it refers to the infringement of the personal autonomy of an incompetent patient. *See* para. 28 *NHS Trust A v M; NHS Trust B v H* [2001] 1 All ER 801.
79 *Ireland v United Kingdom* (1978) 2 EHRR 25.
80 *Herczegfalvy v Austria* (1992) 15 EHRR 437, 484; *T v United Kingdom* (1999) 7 BHRC 659, 682–3.
81 Practice Note (Official Solicitor: Declaratory Proceedings: Medical and Welfare Proceedings for Adults Who Lack Capacity) [2006] 2 F.L.R. 373.
82 Also *Law Hospital NHS Trust v The Lord Advocate* [1996] SLT 848, CT Session (Inner House); *NHS Trust v P* [2000] (Unreported, Dame Elizabeth Butler-Sloss P, 19 December 2000); *Re: H (Adult: Incompetent)* [1998] 2 FLR 36; *Re: D* [1998] 1 FLR 411; *Trust A, Trust B, Dr V v Mr M* [2005] EWHC 807, Fam; *A Hospital v SW* [2007] EWHC 425.
83 Ahsan v University Hospitals Leicester NHS Trust [2006] EWHC 2624.
84 Dyer, C. Withdrawal of food supplement judged as misconduct. *BMJ.* 1999; 318: 895.

19.10.7 The diagnosis is made by reference to the appropriate clinical guidance.[85] Even so, there can be diagnostic doubt in some cases. In *NHS Trust A v H*[86] a 73-year-old woman who had suffered haemorrhagic stroke in 1993 required ANH via PEG feeding to be sustained. P was not diagnosed as being in PVS. She possessed visual tracking and a response to menace. There had been no improvement in her condition after eight years. There was evidence only of fragments of cortical activity. The family and the medical team supported withdrawal of ANH. The Court looked to an *International Working Party Report* [1996] which permitted visual tracking but not focusing on objects or people. The Court concluded that, in fact, P did meet sufficient criteria for PVS and permitted the ANH to be withdrawn. The Royal College of Physicians Guidance was subsequently clarified.[87]

19.10.8 The point here is that the medical complexity in determining a diagnosis and associated prognosis means that they can, and do, fall into issue when dealing with legal questions.

Re: G [1995] 2 FCR 46, Fam

Sir Stephen Brown P

P was a 24-year-old man who was married with a young child. In May 1991, he had been involved in a road traffic accident and suffered head injuries with a subsequent cardiac arrest. In December 1992, P was diagnosed as suffering PVS.

P's wife and D agreed that P's best interests permitted withdrawal of ANH; P's mother disagreed.

Held: Could withdraw feeding.

D had to take into consideration the wishes of the relatives before making the decision, but they were not determinative.

19.10.9 In *Frenchay Healthcare NHS Trust v S*[88] the Court permitted PEG feeding to be withheld in a patient suffering PVS. The initial application was made urgently because the PEG tube had fallen out. An appeal against that decision was lost. Similarly, in the next case, the withholding of

---

85   A report of a working party of the Royal College of Physicians. The vegetative state: guidance on diagnosis and management. *Clin Med.* 2003; **3**: 249–54.
86   [2001] 2 FLR 501, Fam.
87   Dyer, C. Permanent loss of awareness is crucial to diagnosis of PVS. *BMJ.* 2003; **327**: 67.
88   [1994] 2 All ER 403, CA.

ANH by way of not replacing a percutaneous endoscopic gastrostomy (PEG) feeding tube was permitted in another case of PVS.[89]

Swindon & Marlborough NHS Trust v S [1995] 3 Med LR 84, Fam

P was a 48-year-old woman who was being treated for a brainstem tumour. In June 1992, she had surgery. Further surgery to treat a haematoma was complicated by cardiopulmonary arrest. In November 1994, P was diagnosed with PVS.

P was cared for at home and fed via a PEG. The PEG became blocked and an application was made for a declaration that the PEG did not need to be replaced.

Held: The PEG did not need to be replaced.

19.10.10 However, approval to withdraw care has not been given in all cases. In *NHS Trust v J* [90] an application for the withdrawal of ANH in a patient suffering PVS after subarachnoid haemorrhage was deferred so that a therapeutic trial of zolpidem could be undertaken.[91] The option of experimental functional MRI to detect awareness[92] was not accepted as being in the best interests of P by the Official Solicitor. This may have been because the paper was a case report of functional MRI in a single patient.

19.10.11 If awareness could be demonstrated in some cases of PVS then a very difficult situation would arise akin to the situation where the patient suffers a locked-in syndrome. In the only case directly in point, the New Zealand case of *Auckland Area Health Board v A-G*,[93] a 59-year-old man was locked in after suffering Guillain-Barré syndrome. The New Zealand High Court decided that the lack of any chance of recovery permitted the withdrawal of life-preserving treatment. (*See,* also, Section 19.12.4.)

---

89 *Re: M (a minor)* [1998] (Unreported 24 November 1998) – a case of PVS falling directly within the shadow of *Bland*. Permission to withhold artificial feeding and hydration was granted.

90 [2006] EWHC 3152, Fam.

91 *See,* also, *JS v NHS Trust; JA v NHS Trust* [2002] EWHC 2734 where JS was an 18-year-old boy and JA was a 16-year-old girl both suffering variant Creutzfeldt-Jacob disease. The Court approved treatment with an experimental drug Pentosan Polysulphate (PPS).

92 Owen AM, Coleman MR, Boly M, *et al.* Detecting awareness in the vegetative state. *Science.* 2006; **313**(5792): 1402.

93 [1993] 1 NZLR 235.

19.11 FUTILITY BEYOND PVS: ADULTS

19.11.1 The principle of *Bland* applies to all other forms of treatment that might prolong life. Important examples concern respiratory ventilation and do-not-attempt-cardiopulmonary-resuscitation (DNAR) orders. However, these cases are very sensitive to the precise facts of the case.[94] A body of jurisprudence is building from which clear principles are gradually emerging.

19.11.2 A competent patient can determine their own fate (*see* Section 4.5). Therefore, the issues here predominantly surround incompetent adults and children.

NHS Trust v A [2005] EWCA Civ 1145, CA

Waller, Mummery and Tuckey LJJ

P was 86 years old. His past medical history included 1996 CABG, 1999 renal impairment, and stroke disease. Whilst in Pakistan he appeared to have suffered myocardial infarction with acute renal failure and peripheral oedema. He was treated in Islamabad and received at least one cycle of dialysis there.

After discharge, he travelled directly to the UK and went from the airport to a local hospital where he promptly suffered a cardiac arrest. In the intensive care unit he received ventilation, inotropes and renal support inter alia. His transthoracic ECHO revealed only lateral wall motion, implying poor left ventricular function.

P was sentient but incompetent. He struggled against some of the line insertions necessary for his treatment. After a period of time, an initial attempt to withdraw life-sustaining treatment was made with the agreement of the family. Upon withdrawal of care, P improved and was self-ventilating. Active treatment was, therefore, reinstituted. P subsequently deteriorated again.

The medical evidence was that he could survive perhaps six months with intensive-care support, but he was unlikely to become independent ever again and unlikely to regain his competence. The clinicians sought to withdraw life-sustaining care but the family opposed this. The weight of medical evidence was firmly against continuing life-sustaining treatment.

Held: Life-sustaining treatment including ventilation could be withheld. Cardiopulmonary resuscitation could be withheld.

---

94   *Re: K (a minor)* [2006] EWHC 1007, para. 51 per Sir Mark Potter P.

> The Court had to be satisfied to a high degree of probability before it could conclude that life-sustaining treatment was not in the best interests of the patient.

19.11.3 A similar case was *NHS Trust v D*[95] where P was a 32-year-old Roman Catholic woman suffering the late stages of mitochondrial cytopathy. She was unresponsive and, therefore, incompetent. P was self-ventilating via a tracheostomy. She had frequent localised seizures and myoclonic twitching. The medical evidence was that there was no sign of sentience and no hope of recovery. Despite the opposition of the family, the Court concluded that P's best interests did not support continuing active treatment. The medical team were permitted to consider the use of antibiotics if they felt it was appropriate. The aim should be palliation; therefore, mechanical ventilation, cardiopulmonary resuscitation, central venous access and procedures requiring general anaesthesia were precluded.

19.11.4 Life-preserving treatment is not permitted to be withdrawn in all cases. In the next case, the issue was artificial nutrition and hydration in a non-PVS patient. Here the Court chose to continue treatment, basing the decision on the idea that the patient was neither in the dying phase nor was her life intolerable.

W Healthcare NHS Trust v KH [2004] EWCA Civ 1324

P was a 59-year-old woman with multiple sclerosis who required feeding via a percutaneous endoscopic gastrostomy (PEG). P had previously declared that she would not want to be kept alive by machines. Her PEG had fallen out and the issue was whether it should be replaced.

P was conscious but confused. P's family felt that the PEG tube should not be replaced. The medical professionals supported continuing feeding.

Held: PEG should be replaced.

P was not in PVS. Her previous statement was not sufficient to amount to an advance refusal of treatment. Her life was not clearly intolerable. P's best interests lay in continuing her treatment.

---

95 [2005] EWHC 2439, Fam.

19.12 FUTILITY BEYOND PVS: CHILDREN

19.12.1 One situation when the principle of sanctity of life can be overridden by the best interests of the patient is when P's life is 'so demonstrably awful' that treatment could be withheld.[96] In moral terms: a life not worth living, but demonstrably so. The situation must be looked at from the perspective of the patient.

19.12.2 There is a difference between saying that for someone in PVS their interest in living has all but vanished, and a conclusion that a life is so demonstrably awful that efforts to prolong it are not justified. It is here that the arguments in favour of legal recognition of an interest in dying are most powerful. Nevertheless, the glass ceiling of the principle of the sanctity of life remains intact. Therefore active killing is not permissible but the lawful withdrawal of life-sustaining treatment may be possible. In practice, this is simply another flavour of value futility (*see* Section 19.9.2).

19.12.3 The principle was first set out in *Re: B (a minor)(wardship: medical treatment)*.[97] In this case, the surgeon appeared not to be willing to proceed on the basis of the parental refusal of consent; the doctor's reluctance to proceed did not appear to be based on a *bona fide* clinical judgement that the treatment would not benefit the patient.

Re: B (a minor)(wardship: medical treatment) (1981) [1990] 3 ALL ER 927, CA

Templeman, Dunn LJJ

Baby Alexandra case. P suffered trisomy 21 (Down's syndrome) complicated by gastro-intestinal obstruction.[98] The parents refused to consent to surgery. P was made a ward of the court. Initially the court ordered surgery. The surgeon refused to operate in the face of parental refusal of consent.

The evidence was that without surgery the baby would die within three to four days. With surgery, the baby would survive 20 to 30 years, albeit with Down's syndrome.

Held: For surgery, despite the parents' lack of consent.

<u>Templeman LJ:</u> The question to be asked is:

---

96   *Re: C (a minor) (wardship: medical treatment)* [1985] 2 All ER 782, CA.
97   (1981) [1990] 3 All ER 927.
98   ?pyloric stenosis.

'whether the life of this child is demonstrably going to be so awful that in effect the child must be condemned to die, or whether the life of this child is still so imponderable that it would be wrong for her to be condemned to die.'

19.12.4 Whilst formulated in the previous case, this test was applied in the next case.

Re: J (a minor) (wardship: medical treatment) [1990] 3 All ER 930,[99] CA

Ld Donaldson MR, Taylor, Balcombe LJJ

P was a 4½-month-old boy born prematurely at 27 weeks. Birth trauma and prematurity resulted in severe and permanent brain damage. He was very seriously handicapped including spastic quadriplegia, was possibly blind and deaf, and probably had damage to his language centres; he also suffered epilepsy. P could probably feel pain. His life-span was limited significantly by his pathology.

P had required ventilation on several occasions for respiratory arrest. He was at genuine risk of further respiratory arrest. He was off ventilation at the time of trial. Medical opinion was unanimous that the patient should not be for further ventilation.

An application was made for a declaration from the Court that that any further respiratory arrest should not be treated by ventilation, although P should remain for active treatment of infections.

Held: Not-for-ventilation order lawful.

19.12.5 A similar order permitting withholding of mechanical ventilation and other lifesaving treatment was made in *Re: J (a minor) (wardship: medical treatment)*[100] (*see* Section 7.1.15). An important aspect of that case was the point that doctors should not be made to act against their professional judgement.

19.12.6 In the next case, ventilation was withdrawn rather than withheld on similarly tragic facts.

---

99 Wardship points dealt with under consent.
100 [1992] 4 All ER 614.

Re: C (a baby) [1996] 2 FLR 43, Fam

Sir Stephen Brown P

P was a ward of court. She was a 3-month-old baby girl, born eight weeks prematurely, and who suffered neonatal meningitis complicated by severe brain damage about two weeks after birth. She suffered frequent epilepsy and cortical blindness. She was ventilation-dependent and had suffered pain and distress despite having 'very low awareness of anything'.

Medical evidence was that there was no chance of recovery. It was felt that she may survive up to two years on the ventilator, but that she was deteriorating.

Parents, nursing staff and medical opinions were that it was in P's best interests to withdraw ventilation.

Held: Could withdraw ventilation in P's best interests.

19.12.7   Similarly, in *Re: L (a Minor)* [2005] [101] the Court permitted withdrawal of life-preserving treatment including ventilation, despite parental objections, in a child with trisomy 18 (Edward's syndrome). The child had chronic respiratory failure, multiple cardiac defects, epilepsy, severe developmental delay and hypotonia. Full weight was given to 'the child and mankind's desire to survive', [103] but there was no hope of recovery and the treatment was not felt to be promoting any meaningful interests possessed by the child.

19.12.8   Note how these cases contrast with *Bland* where the underlying condition was neither progressive nor fatal. There, the question turned on the value of life without sentience. In both cases, however, the value to the patient of prolonging life was not felt to be sufficient to justify the continuing invasive medical treatment. Here, two principles, futility and a life not worth living, operate in the same direction.

19.12.9   The level of awareness of the patient does not alone determine whether continuing treatment is mandated or not (*see* Section 19.9.1). Compare this next case with the case following (*see* Section 19.12.10).

---

101   *Re: L (a minor)* [2005] 1 FLR 491, Fam, Butler-Sloss P.

Re: C (a minor) (medical treatment) [1998] 1 FLR 384, Fam

Sir Stephen Brown P

P was a 16-month-old girl suffering from spinal muscular atrophy (SMA) type I. She required intermittent positive pressure ventilation, and she had been unable to be weaned from this.

The medical evidence was that SMA type I was a progressive and ultimately fatal condition.

The medical team wanted to wean ventilation because they felt it was futile. The parents were orthodox Jews who, in accordance with their faith, refused consent to withdraw treatment.

Held: Could withdraw ventilation.

Continued ventilation could not be justified in terms of P's best interests. The situation was one of 'No chance' – i.e. where the disease was so severe that life-sustaining treatment delayed death without significant relief of suffering (see Section 19.12.12).

19.12.10 A similar 'No chance' situation arose in *NHS Trust v D*[102] where palliation only was permitted, despite parental objection, for a severely disabled 19-month-old boy who was a ward of court. Because of the fine balance of factors surrounding questions of value futility, withdrawal of ventilation is not always permitted in apparently superficially similar situations.

NHS Trust v MB [2006] EWHC 507, Fam

Holman J

P was an 18-month-old boy who suffered spinal muscular atrophy type I. He also suffered epilepsy. He required intermittent positive pressure ventilation, and he been unable to be weaned from this. P could only move his eyes, the corners of his mouth and thumbs, toes and feet.

The medical evidence was that P could survive for weeks or months, given his condition at that time. There had been a marked deterioration over the last six months. The assumption was that P had normal cognition for his age.

---

102 *NHS Trust v D* [2000] 2 FLR 677.

The medical team sought to withdraw life-preserving treatments, including artificial ventilation. The parents opposed this application. P's Court-appointed Guardian supported the medical position.

Held: It was not in P's best interests to withdraw ventilation. It was not in P's best interests to receive cardiopulmonary resuscitation, ECG monitoring, blood tests or antibiotics.

Here, P might live for up to a year on ventilation and the ventilation could be done via tracheostomy. The need for a 'good death' was not imminent.

The fact of the father's Muslim faith was not relevant to the question of where the child's best interests lay. The fact that the parents actively enriched P's life by maintaining an active relationship and playing him music and DVDs contributed to the positive side of the best interests 'balance sheet'.

19.12.11 This decision can be criticised because it seeks to redraw the distinction between withholding and withdrawing care, a distinction that was rejected by Ld Lowy in *Bland*[68] (*see* Section 19.5.5). However, Holman J made clear that his decision was based in the particular facts of the case and sought to promote the best interests of the child.

19.12.12 In the next case, there was universal agreement that life-prolonging treatment should be withdrawn.

Re: K (a minor) [2006] EWHC 1007, Fam

Sir Mark Potter P

P was a 5½-month-old girl who was born prematurely suffering congenital myotonic dystrophy. Her mother was a sufferer of this condition but the child had a very severe form (genetic anticipation). She was sentient.

Despite aggressive invasive treatment, the child suffered feeding difficulties, progressive muscular weakening and seizures. Gastrointestinal feeding via transpyloric tube had failed, probably because of poor intestinal motility. Therefore, P required central venous access for total parenteral feeding (TPN), with consequent TPN hepatitis and recurrent severe sepsis associated with profound thrombocytopenia.

At the time of application, P was medically stable. The medical evidence was that her prognosis for survival was months at best.

A previous Court order had permitted invasive ventilation and cardiopulmonary resuscitation to be withheld.

Parental responsibility was vested in the Local Authority, not the parents, so an application to the Court was made to permit withdrawal of TPN. All parties agreed that the child's best interests lay in permitting withdrawal of the TPN (line), infusion of fluids and the institution of palliative care.

Held: Withdrawal of TPN permitted, and infusion of fluids for palliative care.

Reference was made to the Royal College of Paediatrics and Child Health guidance: 'Withholding or Withdrawing Life Sustaining Treatment in Children: A Framework for Practice' (2nd Edition), May 2004 and the distinction it drew between a 'No chance' situation and a 'No purpose' situation. It was felt both applied in this case. (*See*, also, *Re: C (a minor) (medical treatment)* [1998], Section 19.12.9.)

The analogy to *NHS Trust v MB*[103] (*see* Section 19.12.10) was considered, but here P could not benefit from external stimulation. Thus, the balance of best interests favoured a different outcome.

19.12.13 This leads to a position where the test of whether a life is 'so demonstrably awful that the child should be condemned to die' (*see* Section 19.12.3) is satisfied when the child can no longer garnish any pleasure from their surroundings and associated stimulation. This must be coupled with no hope of recovery. There is a resonance here with the PVS cases. This situation appears to remove the justification for aggressive invasive measures that potentially cause suffering in such cases.

19.13 CONCLUSION

19.13.1 The end of life raises issues surrounding the culpability of killing or letting die. The interaction between the duty of a medical professional to promote the welfare of their patient and the fact that, in almost all cases, such welfare depends upon continuation of life underpins the principle of the sanctity of life. The principles discussed above look to those few situations where the principle of the sanctity of life is not overriding. These include futile situations, necessary interventions and cases where omissions or unintended consequences are used to exculpate the moral agent.

---

103 [2006] EWHC 507.

Index

DISCOVERY LIBRARY
LEVEL 5 SWCC
DERRIFORD HOSPITAL
DERRIFORD ROAD
PLYMOUTH
PL6 8DH